# SILVER

## NATURE'S
## NATURAL HEALER

Presented by
The Silver Use Institute

Legends
LIBRARY

Published by:

Legends Library Publishing, Inc.

Rochester, NY

www.legendslibrary.org

info@legendslibrary.com

877-222-1960

This is a work of nonfiction. The authors have made every effort to be accurate and complete and welcome comments, suggestions, and corrections, which can be emailed to silveruseinstitute@gmail.com.

All opinions expressed in this work are those of the authors alone.

A free copy of this book is available to read online at silveruseinstitute.com

ISBN-13: 978-1-937735-90-6

Printed in the United States of America

# CONTENTS

Introduction . . . . . . . . . . . . . . . . . . . . . . . . . . . . . . . . . . . . 1

Silver in our Lives . . . . . . . . . . . . . . . . . . . . . . . . . . . . . . . . 1

Why do we need silver supplements, cosmetics and drugs? . . . 2

Very little good information has been available . . . . . . . . . . . 3

My Study of Silver . . . . . . . . . . . . . . . . . . . . . . . . . . . . . . . 3

Different Types of Silver Products . . . . . . . . . . . . . . . . . . . . 4

Ionic Silver Products . . . . . . . . . . . . . . . . . . . . . . . . . . . . . 4

Mild Silver Proteins . . . . . . . . . . . . . . . . . . . . . . . . . . . . . . 5

Old Type Nano Silver Products . . . . . . . . . . . . . . . . . . . . . . 6

Metallic Nano Particle + Ag4O4
(Multiple Modes of Action) . . . . . . . . . . . . . . . . . . . . . . . . . 6

Colloidal Silver . . . . . . . . . . . . . . . . . . . . . . . . . . . . . . . . . 7

Marketing Gibberish . . . . . . . . . . . . . . . . . . . . . . . . . . . . . 7

Particle Size . . . . . . . . . . . . . . . . . . . . . . . . . . . . . . . . . . . 8

Glass vs. Plastic Containers . . . . . . . . . . . . . . . . . . . . . . . . 8

So-Called Alkaline or Structured Silver Products . . . . . . . . . . 9

The Easy Way to Tell if Your Product is
Unique and Superior . . . . . . . . . . . . . . . . . . . . . . . . . . . . . 9

What Is Parts Per Million? . . . . . . . . . . . . . . . . . . . . . . . . . 10

What PPM Silver Supplement Should I Use? . . . . . . . . . . . . . 10

How Much Silver Can I Safely Drink? . . . . . . . . . . . . . . . . . 11

Broad Spectrum Natural Pathogen Killing Machine . . . . . . . . 11

Bacteria Tested and Killed . . . . . . . . . . . . . . . . . . . . . . . . . 12

Yeast, Fungus and Virus Tested and Killed . . . . . . . . . . . . . . 12

Home Brew . . . . . . . . . . . . . . . . . . . . . . . . . . . . . . . . . . . 13

TDS Machines . . . . . . . . . . . . . . . . . . . . . . . . . . . . . . . . . 14

The Problem with Antibiotics . . . . . . . . . . . . . . . . . . . . . . . 14

It Will Get Worse Before It Gets Better . . . . . . . . . . . . . . . . . 14

Toxicity Problem with Antibiotic Usage . . . . . . . . . . . . . . . . 15

Silver May Provide a Ray of Hope . . . . . . . . . . . . . . . . . . . . 16

Not Down On Antibiotics . . . . . . . . . . . . . . . . . . . . . . . . . . 16

Uses of Silver . . . . . . . . . . . . . . . . . . . . . . . . . . . . . . . . . . . 17

Disinfectants. . . . . . . . . . . . . . . . . . . . . . . . . . . . . . . . . . . . 17

Human Studies . . . . . . . . . . . . . . . . . . . . . . . . . . . . . . . . . . . 19

The Safety of Silver Usage . . . . . . . . . . . . . . . . . . . . . . . . . . 19

First-Ever Human Ingestion Study . . . . . . . . . . . . . . . . . . . . 20

Other Silver Safety Studies – Silver Safe for Animals . . . . . . . 20

What is Argyria (The Blue Man Effect)
and How Do You Get It? . . . . . . . . . . . . . . . . . . . . . . . . . . . . 21

Minimum Amount of Silver Intake Known
to Cause Argyria Historically. . . . . . . . . . . . . . . . . . . . . . . . . 22

Colloidal Gold? . . . . . . . . . . . . . . . . . . . . . . . . . . . . . . . . . . . 22

Learning to Use Silver . . . . . . . . . . . . . . . . . . . . . . . . . . . . . . 23

Government Control . . . . . . . . . . . . . . . . . . . . . . . . . . . . . . . . 23

Conclusion . . . . . . . . . . . . . . . . . . . . . . . . . . . . . . . . . . . . . . . 24

Part II General Use Protocols . . . . . . . . . . . . . . . . . . . . . . . . 25

# PART I:
# GENERAL OVERVIEW

## INTRODUCTION

Silver is one of the most beautiful metals that exists. Man has worked for thousands of years to purify and perfect it. Silver is classified as a precious metal, and as such has been highly sought after. "Precious" is a good, descriptive definition of what silver really is. So many people talk about it daily, but so few actually know what it can do. We may have barely begun to scratch the surface in the knowledge of what this beautiful and amazing metal can do to help reduce suffering and possibly save mankind.

Silver has natural, God-given actions unlike any other metal or element that exists. There are many other elements that have value, but none has been blessed with the medicine chest of medicinal effects that silver has. For example, silver has the ability to help with three of the main parts of the body's healing process. First, silver is a natural and very effective antimicrobial. In other words, it can kill a broad spectrum of pathogens like; problem bacteria, yeasts, fungus [5], many parasites [8], and it can even kill or neutralize deadly virus [9][22]. Secondly, silver can help reduce inflammation, and as such can help reduce pain. Third, silver is a natural healing agent, helping the body to create new clean healthy tissue, with reduced scaring [10].

## SILVER IN OUR LIVES

Most people do not know that silver is now used in almost every facet of our modern lives. It is bound to threads that are made into clothes, blankets, bed sheets, etc. The silver kills bacteria that come in contact with the fabric, and it can also kill odor causing bacteria as people work out and sweat. Silver is added to drinks as a colorant and for preservative qualities. Silver is an ingredient in numerous quality cosmetics, for use as a preservative, and also as an active ingredient. Nano silver is imbedded into hundreds of products like washing machines, refrigerators, table tops, cutting boards, handles of all kinds, and steering wheels, to kill bacteria and help keep people from spreading sickness and disease.

Silver is used in almost every electrical connection in every electrical product you own, because it is the number one conductor of both thermal and electrical energy. Its electrical properties also make it a top choice for use in the production of batteries. It can be mixed in with carpet threads, where it is used in expensive computer rooms to reduce static electricity which may damage computers or programs. Silver's superior reflective qualities make it the top choice for the backing of some of the most expensive mirrors. Silver is also used in the production of some of the most expensive quality crystal glassware. Silver is a main ingredient in hundreds of medical products, etc. The list goes on and on and grows almost every day.

## WHY DO WE NEED SILVER SUPPLEMENTS, COSMETICS AND DRUGS?

In the world today we have very few things that can help protect us from invading pathogens that have been able to mutate around the few antibiotics we currently have to fight them. In a report called "The antibiotic crisis", Dr. Arjun Srinivasan of the U.S. CDC was quoted as saying that we may be entering a "post antibiotic era," meaning that deadly pathogens are becoming so resistant to antibiotics that soon they may be of no use at all. Margaret Chan, director-general of the World Health Organization stated, "things as common as strep throat or a child's scratched knee could once again kill."[15] It has already started to happen. A new type of multi-drug resistant bacteria has already entered the U.S. Classified as CRE, these new strains have already traveled through elderly care centers into regular hospitals. According to the U.S. CDC, it is killing over half the people that get infected with it[16]. It is painful to imagine watching family members die from a minor infection that silver could easily treat.

Two published studies already show that silver mixed with antibiotics can make the antibiotics up to hundreds of times more effective, giving new life to antibiotics that have been losing their effectiveness for years.[6][14] The real need now is for us to study and better learn how to use silver to battle these deadly pathogenic problems.

## VERY LITTLE GOOD INFORMATION HAS BEEN AVAILABLE

Until just the last few years the world has been suffering a major knowledge drought about silver and its uses. There has been a great deal of misinformation perpetuated in numerous markets. The good news is that a great deal of very important new scientific information has been published and is readily available on the net for those who wish to have access to the data. For example, one new study showed that mixing silver with antibiotics could make some of the antibiotics as much as 1000 times more effective.[14] That is very important information in a world worried that antibiotics could become useless within just a few years as bacteria continue to mutate and become resistant. Another very important finding was that a new Nano silver was tested in human ingestion studies and shown to have no negative effect when people drank it.[19] [20] This published landmark study showed that when people drank the Nano silver, it hit its highest level or concentration in the blood within two hours and washed out of the body within 24 hours. It was shown that there was no negative effect when people drank the Nano silver liquid, thus dispelling decades of misinformation on how Nano silver might or could be toxic if ingested.

## MY STUDY OF SILVER

I have spent over half of my life studying and working with silver. I have worked for years helping to find it in the ground. I have carefully documented a series of silver veins that run for miles. I have taken a hammer and chisel and have mined it from the veins in the earth, and have crushed it, ground it, and helped melt it into bars. Even with all the time I spent helping a company to amass millions of ounces of silver resources, I had no idea what the real value and what some of the most important uses for silver actually were.

It was not until my father gave me information to read on silver and its therapeutic uses that I began to understand. That information opened a whole new world to me that I did not even know existed. Since that day I have spent thousands of hours studying and seeking real answers to questions about silver. I have studied more than 400 silver reports and studies. I have added value to a number of peer review published articles and studies on some of the medicinal uses of silver. I have been blessed to work with dozens of independent labs, universities, international bio-pharma and government groups, military research groups and hospitals, as well as humanitarian groups, in amassing new knowledge on silver and its abilities. I have been involved in testing and retesting numerous silver products, to come to a better understanding of how and where to use silver to help reduce suffering. I have tried never to accept common knowledge, but to actually work with talented people and labs, to do the test work to prove, and separate out, the fact from the fiction. Along the way, I have been witness to new discoveries and the addition of a significant amount of new knowledge to the world's info base on silver. I wholeheartedly believe that silver is one of God's greatest gifts to us. Silver is a creation that we and our families can learn to use as a first-line-of-defense to help keep our families safe and healthy.

# DIFFERENT TYPES OF SILVER PRODUCTS

There are many different types of silver products; but for the most part there are only three that make up the majority of silver products available on the markets today. Those three are Nano silver products, ionic silver products, and ionic silver protein products. Some types of silver products are useful and some are not very good. Most silver products will actually kill some bacteria and other pathogens, if given a long enough period of time and if they contain a high enough concentration of silver to do so.

# IONIC SILVER PRODUCTS

Ionic Silver is one of the most common forms of silver liquid found in the supplement industry today. Many ionic silver products are made by just diluting chemical forms of silver, like silver nitrate, to a desired use level or parts per million (ppm), which is then bottled and sold to the public. Although ionic silver products have the smallest particle size (which they usually tout), they are often the least stable and can easily fall out of suspension and end up in the bottom of the bottle. Ionic silver products work because each silver ion is missing one electron, which means it has a plus-one charge. The silver ion wants that electron back, so it will steal it from the cell wall of a bacteria for example. When it steals the electron from the cell wall of a bacteria, it pokes a hole in it. If enough silver ions, poke enough holes in the cell wall, then the bacteria dies. But each silver ion can only act or steal an electron once and then it is happy in its state and is of no more use. Because it can only steal one electron before it is neutralized, ionic forms of silver are called *"a one and done technology"*.

Ionic forms of silver are also metabolized, and as a result, in extreme cases where people have consumed large amounts of the product daily over years of use, the silver can build up in the body and cause a condition called argyria. Even with ionic silver products it is very difficult to overdose to the point where you can show symptoms of argyria (blue man look). These ionic silver products are easy to identify because they are often marketed under names like Colloidal silver, Bio Active Silver Hydrosols or Ph Balanced silvers. These products are usually heavily marketed, overpriced, and in the end have very little real substance in the way of individual product testing or information. Their general marketing plans usually take on the motto, "Baffle the public with BS".

## MILD SILVER PROTEINS

Mild silver proteins are simply another form of ionic silver. The only difference is that because ionic forms of silver are not generally stable and because they usually contain large amounts of silver, they sometimes need to be bound to a protein to stay in suspension. The idea behind binding the ionic silver to the protein is to help make the silver stay suspended in the water for longer periods of time. However, as a result of this binding with protein, the silver ions are less functional or useful than traditional ionic silver ions. Consequently, higher levels of silver (ppm) are needed to obtain the desired effect. Sometimes hundreds or even thousands of ppm of silver are added to mild silver protein products to help them be more effective. The producers of these products tout them as being more powerful or effective, because of the higher silver content. In reality they are not, because as stated earlier, the protein inhibits the silver's ability to work. The key to remember with silver proteins is that more silver in a product does not necessarily make it better or more effective.

## OLD TYPE NANO SILVER PRODUCTS

There are some old type Nano silver products on the market, they function much the same way as ionic products. These old products are easy to identify because they are yellow to brown in color. While these products will probably function at some level, they still only have one mode of action. The new improved Nano silver products are clear in color and have multi-action abilities.

## METALLIC NANO PARTICLE + AG4O4 (MULTIPLE MODES OF ACTION)

Metallic Nano forms of silver are by far the most stable form of silver. They are not as easily acted upon by outside forces. They can remain stable for many years and can kill bacteria and other pathogens at very low levels of silver concentration. Nano silver particles can remain stable, because these special Nano particles are coated with a multivalent silver oxide coating or "skin."[4][19] With this outer coating, this new silver particle is attracted to the surrounding water molecules, and as such, becomes semi bound to the structure of the water molecules. This makes the silver much more stable and bioavailable than other types of silver particles. Additionally, the unique Ag4O4 coating gives these silver particles the ability to steal 8 electrons for each silver molecule instead of just one, like regular silver. Each Nano particles is covered with thousands of these super action oxide molecules, making them virtual bacteria or pathogen killing machines.

Studies at some of the top labs in the world have also found that these Nano particles can carry other modes of action as well. These other modes of action include killing pathogens by emitting a resonant frequency. This frequency has been measured to vibrate at between 200–300 nanometers, which is the same vibrational frequency as ultraviolet light. What this means in non-scientific English, is that these particles can put out a wave of energy into water or other liquids, that can kill bacteria and other pathogens that the silver particle doesn't actually have to touch. With these multiple modes of action, silver Nano particles are by far the most effective form of silver that is available on the market.

## COLLOIDAL SILVER

There are many products on the market listed as colloidal silver. In reality the term "colloidal silver" has become so generic that it really means nothing at all. The true definition of colloidal is "particles larger than a molecule in size, suspended in a second solution." This means that only a silver product that is made up of particles that are not too big or too small, and that are suspended in water in a stable manner, could be called a true colloidal silver. The particles have to be larger than a molecule, so that the product can maintain its molecular structure as a metal. Particles that become too small, loose their metallic makeup and become chemical or ionic forms of silver.

An independent group of scientists at Brigham Young University did a study on a number of commercial silver products that were available on the market. All these products claimed to be colloidal silver products. In their report, the group found that almost all of those products were actually just chemical or ionic forms of silver.[1] Further study found that most were very unstable, and that the silver in them could and did fall out of solution or suspension very quickly, ending up as a black residue in the bottom of the container. They also found in comparison tests that the Nano particle products were at least 2–3 times more effective at killing bacteria, than the ionic forms of silver in the commercial colloidal silver products.

## MARKETING GIBBERISH

Many companies that market silver products have no real or useful data on the safety or effectiveness of their products, so they like to argue with each other about two major claims. The first is particle size and the second argument is over the use of glass vs. plastic in the bottling of the products. If you see companies selling silver products, touting or arguing about either of these two items, just know that they probably have no real or useful testing data on their products and that you may want to find another more serious and dedicated company to purchase product from.

## PARTICLE SIZE

As stated earlier, the argument over particle size is mostly one of just marketing gibberish. But that being said, there is a basis for discussion so that you can better understand why the subject is being pushed. The theory behind the argument is that as you break down silver into smaller and smaller particles you increase the surface area. By increasing the surface area, it could increase the effectiveness of the product because there would be more silver exposed to the surrounding environment. That much of the argument is mostly true but only to a point. Other factors have to play in as well. As silver particles are broken down into smaller and smaller particles, they reach a point where they can no longer maintain their molecular structure as a metal and they become ionic or just a single silver ion. Ionic forms of silver are the smallest form of silver available, they are also the most unstable and can easily fall out of solution. They bind with other things like proteins, etc., which mucks up their ability to function and they become a lot less effective. Ionic forms of silver also have only one mode of action, and once used, they become useless (one and done technology—see ionic silver above). So in summary, the smaller the particle size the more silver that is available. But, there is a point where the smaller particle size becomes much less stable, can no longer maintain its molecular structure, and gets bound up, and as such becomes much less useful or effective. So a smaller particle is good but only to a certain point and ionic silver products are past that point.

## GLASS VS. PLASTIC CONTAINERS

Another marketing argument is that silver has to be bottled in glass because plastic containers will negatively affect the silver over time. The statement is just not true. The hard, food grade plastic (PETE) does not negatively affect the silver. In fact, a study completed at BYU, found that glass would sometimes negatively affect silver over time, but the food grade plastic did not.[18] That report also cited two other studies from other independent labs, which found the same thing. So glass could negatively affect the silver, but did not always, but the hard food grade plastic had no negative effect on the silver. The other argument against the hard plastic was that things could possibly leach out of the plastic and into the silver. This was also found to be a false argument.

A study completed on a patented Nano particle liquid silver at Penn State University,[4] found that the silver and also the water were very pure, meaning that no negative elements had leached into the silver liquid from the hard, food grade plastic. Long term stabilities studies also found that Nano silver liquid kept in PET food grade (BPA free) plastic bottles, could easily remain fully active for 7–12 years.

## SO-CALLED ALKALINE OR STRUCTURED SILVER PRODUCTS

These products could best be summarized with the words, disappointing, misrepresented, and with added cold hard lies. I recently found new products listed on the net that claimed to be Alkaline Silver products. The author also claimed the products to be new generation and unique. Upon further investigation I was disappointed to find that most, if not all of the info the doctor was touting, was actually just copies of work from another Nano silver product which the doctor had worked with in the past. For example, numerous pages of cut quotes from the esteemed scientist Dr. Rustum Roy's work was made to look as if it was written about the Alkaline silver product. Unfortunately Dr. Roy had passed away before that product existed, so unless he wrote it from the dead, the work is misrepresented. The doctor also claimed that the competing Nano silver products had acidic Ph.'s of 4.5–5.5, which is just an out-and-out lie. The leading Nano silver products have Ph.'s of between 6.8–7.2, which is almost perfectly neutral, not acidic. The numerous other published reports cited were not from the new product either, but were mixed into his presentations, DVD's, and books to sound like they were. The intent seems to be to deceive the public into thinking his supposedly new product had science behind it. Although very disappointed in his integrity, I understand he is just trying to make a living selling all his relabeled and reshuffled stuff to the public.

## THE EASY WAY TO TELL IF YOUR PRODUCT IS UNIQUE AND SUPERIOR

The easy way to tell if you have a superior product or a mediocre one is to check the label on the product or box for patent numbers. US Patents are only granted to products that prove they are different and unique from all others on the market. If your silver product is patented it means that your product proved by hard science to the US Government that it was different and unique from all others. It is the only way to know for sure that your silver product is not just another form of the same old stuff. Check the label. If a product is patented it will give the patent number on the label. Once you have that number you can go to the US Patent website and put in that number and be able to pull up the patent and read it. Claims and tests used to prove the uniqueness of the product will be listed in the patents. A little bit of diligence on your part in looking up the patent number, may open up a whole new world of information to you.

## WHAT IS PARTS PER MILLION?

Silver content in supplement products is usually stated as "parts per million," or "ppm." The term parts per million is really pretty easy to understand. If a product's label states that it has a 10 ppm silver content, this means that for every million parts water, there are 10 parts of silver. It does not mean that there are only 10 little pieces of silver in the bottle. It means that if you added up all the silver particles together, there would be 10 parts of silver for every million parts of water. In other words, a very small amount of silver can usually do some really amazing things.

## WHAT PPM SILVER SUPPLEMENT SHOULD I USE?

After years of study I believe that the best products to use on a daily basis are between 10–20 ppm of a patented Nano silver product. If there is a greater need I would use products up to a range of maybe 30 ppm. Never use a product with high ppm content, it is not needed nor safe no matter what the salesman may claim, even if the salesman claims he is also a doctor. Drinking a 200 ppm product for example, is like cleaning snow off your driveway with a bulldozer. It would probably work, but the damage a bulldozer could do to your driveway would be severe. The claim is usually that these high ppm products kill bacteria in test tubes very fast, Clorox also kills surface bacteria fast but I would not recommend drinking that either. What is needed is a level of silver strong enough to kill pathogenic bacteria but also safe enough not to kill probiotic or good bacteria (helpful bacteria used in digestion). I have access to hundreds of studies, which cost millions of dollars to complete, which I used to help determine what the optimum silver levels are to use internally. Testing I have personally seen shows that so called colloidal or ionic silver products sold at levels between 100 and two 200 ppm or higher are not safe for internal human use, they kill not only the bad bacteria but also the good. A 100–200 ppm silver product can also kill an excessive amount of regular human cells (called cytotoxicity). Do not drink them they are not safe. In summary use only good quality Nano silver products at silver levels between 10 and 30 ppm.

## HOW MUCH SILVER CAN I SAFELY DRINK?

The US EPA is the governing body when it comes to toxicity of most products. In a document called the RED document (Registration Eligibility Document)[3] on page two, the document states that the daily recommended intake limit on silver is .005/mg/kg. What that means in English, is that by government standards, an average sized adult could safely drink up to an ounce (six teaspoons) of a 10 ppm silver product every day for their entire life, and that amount would be deemed safe by U.S. EPA standards. The document goes on to state (page 4, 4th paragraph) that the EPA does not anticipate that dietary exposure to these low levels of silver will be associated with any significant degree of risk. Another study found that human ingestion of the Nano silver liquid at both 10 and 32 ppm had no negative effect on any tested system in the body.[19]

## BROAD SPECTRUM NATURAL PATHOGEN KILLING MACHINE

Silver is one of the most broad-spectrum antimicrobial elements that exists. Broad spectrum means that silver can kill a wide variety of pathogens. Silver will kill bad or harmful bacteria, fungus, yeast, and mold, neutralize virus, and also a number of protozoa. The ability to kill such a variety of bad bugs, is very unique. An antibiotic for example, that you may get from a doctor, may have the ability to kill a few different kinds of bacteria, like a type called "gram negative", but most often it will be limited to just one or two types of bacteria. Antibiotics cannot usually kill a bad type of yeast, like candida, and will certainly not kill or neutralize a virus that causes the flu. Nano silver, on the other hand, can not only kill a large variety of bacteria, yeast, fungus, virus and other pathogens, but it can do it without damaging the human or animal using it. It is truly a gift to the person who knows how to use it.

## BACTERIA TESTED AND KILLED

Numerous tests have proven that Nano silver in very small quantities can kill numerous deadly forms of bacteria like MRSA (a multi- drug resistant form of staph infection that kills tens-of-thousands of people annually).[24] A person can be infected with the MRSA form of staph infection at a baseball field, gym, locker room, bathroom, playground, park bench, waiting room, kitchen, restaurant, airplane etc. etc. It is one of the most deadly bacteria that infects people in U.S. hospitals. Testing has also proven that Nano silver will kill numerous other deadly forms of bacteria as well. Bacteria like: Anthrax; Tuberculosis (the number one cause of death by infection on the earth right now); food poisoning bacteria like E. coli (the culprit bacteria in most food poisoning cases that sooner or later we all get) and Salmonella; Y. pestis (the bacteria that causes Bubonic Plague[21] or black death, which killed tens of millions of people in Europe); H. influenza; and numerous different strains of streptococcus; and many other pathogenic bacteria too numerous to list here.

## YEAST, FUNGUS AND VIRUS TESTED AND KILLED

Testing has also proven that silver Nano-particles, in the right form, kill pathogenic yeasts, like Candida yeast.[25] Candida causes problems like vaginal yeast infections, the worst types of diaper rash and a number of other common problems. Silver Nano-particles can also kill or neutralize virus like Hepatitis C., SARS, Beijing flu, three different types of Bird flu including the deadly H5–N1 type.[9] Test work has proven that silver Nano-particles will kill different kinds of mold and environmental fungus like black mold.[26] Black mold plagues many houses and office buildings in the United States, causing upper and lower-respiratory-tract infections among family members and employees. The fact is that in test-tube testing, not one pathogenic (bad or deadly) organism has been tested that could not be killed with small amounts of engineered silver Nano-particles.

# HOME BREW

Many people say that they do not need to buy a silver product because they have a little machine at home that will make it for pennies per gallon. I usually ask them if they also go yank willow bark off of a tree and chew it when they have a headache. White willow bark is used to make aspirin. The point is that when they make that product in their house, they have no idea what they are making or drinking. It could have one part per million silver or 10,000 parts per million. There is really no way to know with any assurance, unless you tested each and every batch of product that was made, using an AA (atomic absorption) or equivalent type of machine. An AA machine can measure silver levels in liquid in parts per million or even parts per billion. A group I personally know, found in testing the home-brew machines that the products made by them would be vastly different every single time product was made. This is true even if a person uses the same water, the same silver, and makes the product for the exact same period of time, each time product is made.

The silver product made by "home-brew" machines can be of very poor quality. There are a number of other problems with these machines. The first problem is that the particles that these machines make are usually too big to enter into the human system, and thus are mostly ineffective. The second problem is that because the products are so ineffective, the people who use them usually have to drink a lot of the product to get a positive reaction. Third, the increased amount of home-brew product needed to get a good reaction is usually way above what a person should safely drink on a daily basis. When people drink large amounts of heavy or loaded home-brew silver products, they potentially expose themselves to a condition called argyria. (I will give more information on this condition in the safety section). I have searched and there just isn't a good way to accurately and cheaply measure silver content in home-brew products. I do however think that the home-brew products are good for one thing, and that is to kill infection on the outside of the body. The bigger particles that these home brew machines make, I believe, can safely disinfect wounds, burns, and cuts outside the body without causing any problems, but my advice is that you do not drink them in any large quantity.

## TDS MACHINES

TDS stands for "total dissolved solids". These small hand held devices are really no more than toys. They do not measure silver alone but supposedly every dissolved element contained in the water, it can make no distinction as to what is in the water, just that something is dissolved in it. The problem is that these small, inexpensive devices are not very accurate, a simple change in the water temperature is enough to change what the machine reads as total dissolved solids in the water, sometimes by 100's of percentage points. If you realize that these machines are not very accurate, then it is fine to use one. If you intend to get an accurate reading on the amount of silver contained in any silver water, you must use an AA Machine (atomic absorption) or the equivalent. These machines however are expensive, but they can accurately read silver content in water to parts per billion, not to just parts per million.

## THE PROBLEM WITH ANTIBIOTICS

Silver is gaining popularity because antibiotics are failing to get the job done. In fact, we are at a point where we are being attacked from all sides with deadly bacteria and virus. Our antibiotic guns are falling further and further short of their targets. We are obviously under the constant threat of bio-weapons, but the real threat to your family may be the local school yard or your neighborhood hospital. The problem is real, and as hundreds of thousands of people can attest, *deadly*. The problem has become so bad that some people are now refusing to go to local hospitals for needed treatment, because they are afraid of coming in contact with a bacterial pathogen that antibiotics cannot stop and which may actually kill them.[15] A friend in Virginia told me of one of his neighbors who had fallen off his barn roof and broken his ankle, a compound fracture. He had gone to the hospital where they had routinely reset his ankle and sent him home. He was dead three days later from a staph infection he had acquired while in the hospital having his ankle treated.

## IT WILL GET WORSE BEFORE IT GETS BETTER

This death of a neighbor is not an isolated case, and as bacterial resistance continues to grow rampant, it will become more and more common, affecting our friends, neighbors and even our own children. I can think of no greater hell than to watch helplessly as a loved one dies because of antibiotic resistant bacteria, after everything in the doctors' prescription arsenal has been tried and failed. When talking about antibiotic resistance with Forbes Magazine (Bug Wars, July 7th, 2003 pg.137), Hank A. McKinnell, Chief executive of Pfizer stated, "There are a number of organisms where we're one antibiotic away from a world-wide disaster." Think of it, unstoppable plague-like bacterial infections that could kill millions. It has happened before. The Forbes article also goes on to state, "Drug resistant strains of everything from tuberculosis to staphylococcus are killing tens of thousands of patients every year. Penicillin is now useless against one third of all Streptococcus pneumonia, a common cause of pneumonia, meningitis and ear infections."

## TOXICITY PROBLEM WITH ANTIBIOTIC USAGE

Another real problem we face as consumers and parents is that most of the antibiotics we have left in our arsenal to use against sickness are very toxic, not only to bacteria but also to us. Antibiotics often have serious side effects, including changes in heart rhythm, liver toxicity and even death. Barbara Starfield, in a December 2000, Journal of the American Medical Association article, stated that an estimated 106,000 people had died that year as a side effect of antibiotics used "correctly". That number did not include people who died because of antibiotics given in error or in a bad combination, or people who had been maimed but who had not died, but only people who had died as a direct side effect of antibiotics that were used correctly! The problem with this is that death is a very permanent side effect! We went to war in Afghanistan because the Taliban had killed a total of about 3,000 people in the twin towers. The September 11th terrorist attacks were, in fact, a terrible tragedy. When you consider, however, the fact that antibiotics (used correctly) killed an estimated 42 times that many people in just one year, you will realize that the number of people killed on 9/11 is only a drop in the bucket when compared to the number of people killed annually as a side effect of using prescription antibiotics. In all my years of study, I have never found even one case of a person who died as a result of the medicinal use of silver supplement products.

## SILVER MAY PROVIDE A RAY OF HOPE

With the fact that pharmaceutical companies have only come up with one new class of bacteria- fighting antibiotics in the last 35 years (Pfizer's Zyvox), it would seem that the new hope for our survival will have to come from elsewhere. Many pharmaceutical companies are now spending their time just reworking, or selling at stronger levels (which increases the negative side effects), antibiotics that have been on the market for years, hoping that they can both buy time and sustain their bottom-line financial profits. Time currently does not seem to be on their side.

A natural answer to this problem may be the use of silver. Silver was heavily used to treat disease before the advent of antibiotics. Various forms of silver have been used for years in the medical industry. In fact, there are over eighty products currently approved or cleared by the U.S. FDA that are based on silver and its ability to kill bad bugs.[27] Not only that, but one published study out of BYU[5] showed that Nano silver was as effective or more effective than numerous forms of antibiotics. Another study showed that Nano silver did not promote resistance in bacteria strains, because of multiple modes of killing actions and broad spectrum of antimicrobial abilities, meaning that the Nano silver had a number of different ways to kill many different types of harmful bacteria etc., where regular antibiotics did not.[29]

## NOT DOWN ON ANTIBIOTICS

I want you to know that I am not an extremist and I do not believe that silver will cure every disease that plagues mankind with ease. I do believe that silver is our best first-line-of-defense, saving antibiotics for those rare times when they may really be needed. Most pathogenic problems are easily solved with silver, when a person gains a knowledge of how to use it. But, when death of a loved one is on the line because of a disease or infection, sometimes it is time to pull out all the stops and really attack the problem.

One scientific report[6] goes one step further. It is a report where testing was done using Nano silver along with antibiotics, to make the antibiotics more effective. This report found that silver had an added value to all of the 19 antibiotics tested. This means that in the most difficult cases, it may be best to double up on the disease or infection by using both antibiotics and the silver product at the same time. This may better appease the mainstream medical community, and at the same time save the lives of many people. I am aware of one case of a woman patient in a military hospital, who had been on antibiotics for a number of months to try to eliminate a drug resistant E. coli infection in her urinary tract. The months of treatment with antibiotics were unable to help her eliminate the problem. The woman was suffering from a great deal of pain and discomfort because of the infection. The doctor then used a 10 ppm Nano silver supplement in combination with the drugs and the patient was able to fully recover and leave the hospital within two weeks. The doctor shortly thereafter was so impressed with the added action of the silver, that she gave the person who sent her the silver product a big hug and called him an "angel of mercy". A brand new study by Boston University also came to the same conclusion, finding that silver could make the antibiotics as much as 1000 times more effective.[14]

## USES OF SILVER

Nano silver is not only good for use as a first-line-of-defense and antibiotic alternative supplement and wound healer, but it can also be used as a very important personal disinfectant. It can be used as a safe disinfectant for people, places and things. Each of these usage areas are vast and very important.

## DISINFECTANTS

Silver is uniquely useful as a disinfectant. As previously stated, one of the major problems in the world today is the number of deadly pathogens that have mutated to the point were few things can kill them. Most of the disinfectants designed to kill these "super bugs" are themselves so toxic that they can kill or maim children who accidently handle, drink, or sometimes even just come in contact with them. People often use very poisonous disinfectants in bathrooms, on counter tops and refrigerator handles, even on floors that our kids may crawl on.

If we use these products around our families, sooner or later, these poisons may enter into our children's mouths. It may be true that these poisons may not kill our children quickly, although they certainly can. But how many children do you know that have contracted cancer or some other strange disease. These strange diseases are becoming very common-place and more and more children seem to be affected by them. I am not pointing a finger, only asking a question about the possible end result of being contaminated time and time again by disinfectant poisons.

Nano silver, in contrast, when used in the right form, can become a "super disinfectant," one that is non-toxic to both adults and children. It is not quite as fast as chemical disinfectants, killing most problem bacteria in about 2-15 minutes, where most of the nasty chemical disinfectants will kill the bacteria in seconds. The important fact is that Nano silver products used in small amounts can safely disinfect areas were people live and work, and were children play. They can be made to be so pow-erful that they can be used to disinfect hospital operating rooms, and at the same time so safe that if your child were to accidently drink a whole bottle, he or she would suffer no ill effects. They can be used where other disinfectants cannot, like in disinfecting a child's wheelchair with him/her still in it, or disinfecting a baby's crib without removing the baby. A person would never want to use chemical disinfectants to disinfectant children's toys for example, but silver would be safe to use on them.

Silver disinfectants can be made with no color, smell or chemicals ad-ditives, unlike other disinfectant products. Nano-particle silver products will not burn the skin, or even leave your house smelling like a hospital or dental office. In tests for homeland defense, an engineered silver Nano-particle disinfectant product was able to kill 81,000,000 Bubonic Plague bacteria, in less than two minutes of contact time.[21] This proves that silver products, made carefully and in a highly controlled way, can, in fact, eliminate pathogens that could potentially kill millions of people, and can do it in a way that presents no danger to humans.

Silver however, should only be used on non-porous surfaces (surfaces without microscopic holes in them) because if it gets in small cracks or holes and dries there, it can cause some discoloration of the surface ma-terial over time. The discoloration will be a greyish color, so it would not be a problem for darker surfaces, but it may be for light colors.

## HUMAN STUDIES

One of the things that has been lacking in the use of silver supplement products, is the actual proof that they can help people when they are used internally. There are multitudes of claims that have been and are being made, by tens of thousands people, each giving their own personal stories, but real medical studies have been lacking. A group of people wanted to see if silver products would actually help people in hospitals in Africa. Silver supplement products were donated so that the African people could do their own tests. These African people tested the products in 124 cases in four different hospitals and clinics in Ghana, West Africa. The people wanted to see if silver, working jointly with the immune system could help people get better.

In the studies, the 10 ppm engineered silver-Nano-particle supplement product was tested as an alternative to the antibiotics in 18 different types of human problems. The studies tested the product's ability to treat conditions such as nasal infections, eye infections, sore throats, cuts, urinary tract infections, ear infections, bronchitis, upper respiratory tract infections, malaria and gonorrhea, etc. The product was used both internally and externally. In the entire study there were no treatment failures, and almost every patient was in full recovery within just 7 days.

The product was proven effective in helping to alleviate all 18 human ailments tested. The Food and Drug Board of Ghana awarded the engineered silver-nano-particle product a drug approval as a homeopathic drug. Three additional human studies have been completed for a total of 124 patients. What has been proven in the human case studies is that Nano silver can, in fact, help people to overcome numerous human ailments as an effective immune enhancing product. The information from this testing was released to the public by the US Congress, in the form of a US Congressional Testimony.[17]

## THE SAFETY OF SILVER USAGE

Silver, when used in small amounts is non-toxic to humans. It can be used every day if taken at safe levels. The standard for the amount of silver that can be safely consumed daily in water, was established by the United States EPA. The EPA established the Reference Dose (RfD) or daily intake limit, in 1991. It established the amount of silver that can be safely consumed daily at .005 milligrams per kilogram of body weight per day (EPA RED document on silver page 2, 4th paragraph). What that means, simply, is that a normal sized adult, could safely consume one ounce (6 tsp) of a 10 PPM silver product every day, for a 72 year life span and still be within the safe limits as defined by the EPA. In the EPA RED document for silver, the EPA goes on to state (3rd page, 4th paragraph), "The EPA does not anticipate that dietary exposure to these low levels of silver, will be associated with any significant degree of risk." The one ounce per day safety level corresponds directly with the amount of the silver product that was used in the hospital studies in Africa. In those studies, the doctors were using up to 6 teaspoons daily (one ounce) to successfully help treat the human ailments.

## FIRST-EVER HUMAN INGESTION STUDY

In 2013, a ground breaking new study was completed and published. This new study was the first ever single blind human ingestion study on silver ever completed in the history of the world.[19] The study tested the safety of humans drinking engineered silver Nano particle supplement products at both 10 and 32 ppm. The 60 people drank about 3 teaspoons of the silver products daily for 14 days. The study concluded that drinking either the 10 or 32 ppm silver Nano particle supplements had no negative effect on any system in the body. It was also found that after drinking the products, the silver hit its high point in the blood in about two hours, and the Nano silver washed out of the body in about 24 hours. The human study also covered checking the blood platelet cells for any negative action. It was found that the silver had no negative action or effect on the blood cells.[20] Both of these human ingestion studies have been peer reviewed and published and are currently available in PubMed.

## OTHER SILVER SAFETY STUDIES – SILVER SAFE FOR ANIMALS

Other completed safety studies include in vivo (living) toxicity tests completed on silver products. In the animal tests, the products were tested at as much as 200 times the normal adult dosage, or a level equivalent to a human adult consuming or drinking about 32 full ounces of 10 ppm silver product at one sitting.[12] At the conclusion of the tests, the independent lab reported that the product was found completely non-toxic to the test animals at that high level of consumption. Two other independent cytotoxicity tests have been completed on both a 10 and a 22 ppm supplement product. In these tests, both products were tested for toxicity in both human epithelial and African green monkey cells. At the conclusion of the tests, the lab reported, "Cell lines treated with the 10 and 22 ppm silver products were indistinguishable from the control indicating no cytotoxicity."[28] In other words, the silver did not harm the human or monkey cells at all. Also, both injected and ingested tests have been completed on animals at levels of up to 5,000 milligrams per kilogram of body weight[11] (a lot of silver taken at one time), and those tests found that the silver products, even at levels of up to 32 ppm, were completely non-toxic to the test animals. These tests show that animals can also be given the Nano silver supplements to help support their immune systems, and even at very high levels of ingested silver, the silver will not hurt the animals.

## WHAT IS ARGYRIA (THE BLUE MAN EFFECT) AND HOW DO YOU GET IT?

Argyria, also known as the blue man syndrome, has resulted from the extreme misuse of very strong silver solutions. It is caused by people drinking large amounts of ionic silver products over years and years of misuse. It cannot come from the ordinary use of supplemental silver products. Most of the cases I have seen, have been from people making their own products at home with a cheap generator, then drinking 20–30 ounces daily over a period of years. It is not easy to get argyria. Even with ionic silver products, they wash out of your system fairly quickly. In order to get argyria you have to drink so much silver that your body cannot wash it out fast enough. When you get an excess of silver in your body, your body will try to get rid of the excess silver by walling it off in your cells. It is like a tattoo of silver under your skin. Like a tattoo, it has no negative effect except it discolors your skin. Once you expose this silver to sunlight, the silver oxidizes and the skin turns grey. It is a permanent condition like a tattoo. Rustum Roy, the famed material scientist, explained in one of his published scientific papers on silver that argyria can only come from ionic forms of silver.[4] You cannot get it from metallic nano particles. The believed reason is that the Nano forms of silver are not metabolized and are washed out of the body too quickly, so they cannot build up in the system. This theory is also backed by the human ingestion safety study as outlined above.[19]

## MINIMUM AMOUNT OF SILVER INTAKE KNOWN TO CAUSE ARGYRIA HISTORICALLY

For those people who are really worried about the subject of argyria, a little more information may be important. Hill and Pillsbury (1939) stated, "The ordinary clinical use of silver compounds practically never gives rise to any gross untoward effect other than argyria." The minimum amount of silver known to cause argyria in adults, from the use of any silver compound (including ionic salts) is 900 mg of silver taken orally in one year. In order to reach this level of silver intake, an individual would have to consume at least 380–8 oz. bottles of a 10 PPM silver product within a year. Most suggested adult dosages are about ½ to 1 teaspoon taken one to three times daily. This means that an individual would have to consume over 50 times the normal adult dosage, every day for a year to even reach the lowest level ever known to cause argyria. It should be noted that EPA standards for the amount of silver that can be safely consumed in drinking water is about one ounce a day of a 10 ppm product, as stated earlier.[3] In other words, using silver daily in small dosages as a supplement really has no negative risk associated with it.

## COLLOIDAL GOLD?

Some people think that since we use silver as a natural healer and pathogen killer, that we should also eat or drink colloidal gold. I have studied it for years and my family actually owns mines that produce gold. For that reason, I would love to tell you that I have found value in consuming gold, but I have not. Unlike silver, gold is a heavy metal and if you eat it, it can cause damage to your kidneys.[2] The term is called heavy metal poisoning or toxic nephropathy. Gold is not a healing agent and it is also not a bacteria or pathogen killing machine like silver is. So in summary, gold is cool and pretty, but it can be toxic if you eat or drink it. There is good reason why silver has been used for centuries as a medicinal metal and gold has not.

# LEARNING TO USE SILVER

The greatest weakness when it comes to using silver is not that it cannot work to reduce the suffering of millions of people. The weakness is actually ours, in the fact that we need to increase our knowledge to help us learn how to better utilize this gift from God. As we increase our knowledge, we will increase our ability to reduce the pain and suffering of many people worldwide. Remember, what effects one, can and will affect all of us at some point in time.

# GOVERNMENT CONTROL

I have been amazed lately at what seems to be an extreme bias against Nano silver liquid products by many governments and so called health groups, especially in light of its ability to work with low cost and without the harsh side effects of most antibiotics and other drugs. I believe that most government agencies have enough information available to know that it can help to relieve many problems. I have come to the conclusion that they could care less about saving lives or reducing pain, the bias is more about control and money. It seems that a good worldwide pandemic (world spreading of a deadly disease) is what they hope for so that they can fill their accounts with money to fight it. If it did not happen or if it could be solved easily with a natural product, they would not get the money they want. So they push the use of drugs they cannot supply so that the problem can get worse quickly. It is like they want to keep telling people the world is flat, so that people will not leave the area for fear of falling off the edge.

When people come to know what Nano silver can do for them and their families, dependence on some government agencies will be much reduced. This will also reduce the need for many expensive antibiotics and other drugs, whose companies contribute money to those political groups and organizations. Truth always has a way of coming out in the end and lives will be saved in spite of so called government health groups. The earth is not flat and I know that Nano silver can and will do many things to save lives and help reduce the suffering of people around the world.

## CONCLUSION

Silver is one of the greatest medicinal gifts that God has given mankind. Silver has many attributes that make it effective in helping to keep mankind safe and healthy. First, silver is a very effective broad-spectrum antimicrobial agent, meaning that it can kill many different types of problem bacteria, yeast, fungus, parasites, and it can neutralize virus. Second, a great deal of mounting evidence suggests that silver is also a very effective anti-inflammatory agent, meaning that it can reduce inflammation and pain in the body. Third, Nano silver is also a healing agent that can help wounds heal that will not normally heal. It also helps to heal regular wounds in about half the normal time. So in essence, silver, in small amounts, has the ability to help treat infections, mitigate disease, and reduce the suffering of millions of people. There are many different types of silver products on the market, and there is a huge difference in the effectiveness of these different types of silver products. Used at low silver levels, Nano silver is the most effective type of silver technology on the market today. We need to come to a better understanding and knowledge of how to utilize silver to further reduce suffering worldwide.

# Part II:
# General Use
# Protocol
# Suggestions

## NANO SILVER GEL AND LIQUID GENERAL USE SUGGESTIONS

Every person's body is different, every case is different, and there are no one-size-fits-all treatment protocols. For that reason, the protocols listed herein are to be considered general use suggestions only. For serious health problems always consult your physician! For most general internal use purposes, I suggest the use of a 10 ppm Nano silver liquid product. A good quality Nano silver 10 ppm product is safe for everyday use and will have the ability to help handle most problems. A slightly higher ppm Nano silver product (up to an 18 to 32 ppm) has also been shown to also be safe in a published human ingestion study when used on a daily basis.[19] I suggest use of the higher ppm only if a person feels that they just need a little extra help in supporting the immune system. A quality 24 ppm Nano silver gel product is also usually more than enough to help solve most external infection or skin irritation problems. I do not recommend the use of silver products over about 35 ppm. The fact is that you can only kill bacteria and other pathogens so dead, and the use of higher silver levels does not make them any more dead. Overuse of high ppm ionic products can cause the condition argyria. Also remember that no element or product is perfect for all situations, but Nano silver is amazingly good in many situations!

## SPECIFIC CONDITIONS TREATED

Nano Silver Gel and Liquid General Use Suggestions. . . . . . .25

Specific Conditions Treated. . . . . . . . . . . . . . . . . . . . . . . . . .26

Abdominal Pain & Diarrhea . . . . . . . . . . . . . . . . . . . . . . . . .29

Acne . . . . . . . . . . . . . . . . . . . . . . . . . . . . . . . . . . . . . . . . . . .29

AIDS. . . . . . . . . . . . . . . . . . . . . . . . . . . . . . . . . . . . . . . . . . .30

Allergies . . . . . . . . . . . . . . . . . . . . . . . . . . . . . . . . . . . . . . . .30

Animal Uses . . . . . . . . . . . . . . . . . . . . . . . . . . . . . . . . . . . . .30

Antibiotic Use . . . . . . . . . . . . . . . . . . . . . . . . . . . . . . . . . . .30

Asthma . . . . . . . . . . . . . . . . . . . . . . . . . . . . . . . . . . . . . . . . .31

Athlete's Foot . . . . . . . . . . . . . . . . . . . . . . . . . . . . . . . . . . . .31

Bedsores . . . . . . . . . . . . . . . . . . . . . . . . . . . . . . . . . . . . . . . .32

Bird Flu. . . . . . . . . . . . . . . . . . . . . . . . . . . . . . . . . . . . . . . . .32

Black Mold . . . . . . . . . . . . . . . . . . . . . . . . . . . . . . . . . . . . . .33

Body Odor . . . . . . . . . . . . . . . . . . . . . . . . . . . . . . . . . . . . . .34

Bronchitis . . . . . . . . . . . . . . . . . . . . . . . . . . . . . . . . . . . . . . .34

Bug Bites/Spider Bites. . . . . . . . . . . . . . . . . . . . . . . . . . . . . .34

Burns & Cuts . . . . . . . . . . . . . . . . . . . . . . . . . . . . . . . . . . . .35

Cancers . . . . . . . . . . . . . . . . . . . . . . . . . . . . . . . . . . . . . . . . .36

Cankers & Other Mouth Sores . . . . . . . . . . . . . . . . . . . . . . .39

Chicken Pox . . . . . . . . . . . . . . . . . . . . . . . . . . . . . . . . . . . . .39

Cold Sores . . . . . . . . . . . . . . . . . . . . . . . . . . . . . . . . . . . . . .40

Common Colds . . . . . . . . . . . . . . . . . . . . . . . . . . . . . . . . . . .40

Dandruff . . . . . . . . . . . . . . . . . . . . . . . . . . . . . . . . . . . . . . . .40

Dental Applications . . . . . . . . . . . . . . . . . . . . . . . . . . . . . . .41

Diabetic Neuropathy (Sores). . . . . . . . . . . . . . . . . . . . . . . . .42

Diaper and Other Rashes . . . . . . . . . . . . . . . . . . . . . . . . . . .43

Disinfection of Cutting Boards. . . . . . . . . . . . . . . . . . . . . . .44

Ear Aches both Internal And External. . . . . . . . . . . . . . . . . .44

EBOLA . . . . . . . . . . . . . . . . . . . . . . . . . . . . . . . . . . . . . . . . .45

Eczema . . . . . . . . . . . . . . . . . . . . . . . . . . . . . . . . . . . . . . . . .46

# PART II: GENERAL USE PROTOCOL SUGGESTIONS

Emergency Storage . . . . . . . . . . . . . . . . . . . . . . . . . . . . . . .46

Eye Infections . . . . . . . . . . . . . . . . . . . . . . . . . . . . . . . . . .47

Eye (Tired Eyes). . . . . . . . . . . . . . . . . . . . . . . . . . . . . . . . .48

Facials . . . . . . . . . . . . . . . . . . . . . . . . . . . . . . . . . . . . . . .48

Flu. . . . . . . . . . . . . . . . . . . . . . . . . . . . . . . . . . . . . . . . . .49

Food Poisoning . . . . . . . . . . . . . . . . . . . . . . . . . . . . . . . . .49

Fungal / Yeast Skin Infections . . . . . . . . . . . . . . . . . . . . . . .50

Fungus Infections of the Feet: . . . . . . . . . . . . . . . . . . . . . . .50

General Well-being . . . . . . . . . . . . . . . . . . . . . . . . . . . . . . .51

Gingivitis. . . . . . . . . . . . . . . . . . . . . . . . . . . . . . . . . . . . . .51

Gonorrhea . . . . . . . . . . . . . . . . . . . . . . . . . . . . . . . . . . . . .52

Hand Sanitizer . . . . . . . . . . . . . . . . . . . . . . . . . . . . . . . . . .52

Hair Gel and Head Rub. . . . . . . . . . . . . . . . . . . . . . . . . . . .53

Hemorrhoids . . . . . . . . . . . . . . . . . . . . . . . . . . . . . . . . . . .53

Hepatitis B/C. . . . . . . . . . . . . . . . . . . . . . . . . . . . . . . . . . .53

HIV (AIDS) . . . . . . . . . . . . . . . . . . . . . . . . . . . . . . . . . . . .55

HPV (Vaginal Papilloma Virus Infection). . . . . . . . . . . . . . . .56

Inflammation of the Joints:. . . . . . . . . . . . . . . . . . . . . . . . . .57

Injection and IV Therapy . . . . . . . . . . . . . . . . . . . . . . . . . . .58

Itch . . . . . . . . . . . . . . . . . . . . . . . . . . . . . . . . . . . . . . . . . .58

Jelly Fish Sting . . . . . . . . . . . . . . . . . . . . . . . . . . . . . . . . . .59

Jock Itch . . . . . . . . . . . . . . . . . . . . . . . . . . . . . . . . . . . . . .59

Laryngitis . . . . . . . . . . . . . . . . . . . . . . . . . . . . . . . . . . . . . .59

Liver Problems. . . . . . . . . . . . . . . . . . . . . . . . . . . . . . . . . . .59

Lyme Disease . . . . . . . . . . . . . . . . . . . . . . . . . . . . . . . . . . .60

Malaria . . . . . . . . . . . . . . . . . . . . . . . . . . . . . . . . . . . . . . .61

Massage Therapy . . . . . . . . . . . . . . . . . . . . . . . . . . . . . . . .62

Mastitis . . . . . . . . . . . . . . . . . . . . . . . . . . . . . . . . . . . . . . .62

Molds and Environmental Fungi . . . . . . . . . . . . . . . . . . . . . .63

Mouth Wash. . . . . . . . . . . . . . . . . . . . . . . . . . . . . . . . . . . .63

Periodontal Disease . . . . . . . . . . . . . . . . . . . . . . . . . . . . . . .63

Personal Lubricant. . . . . . . . . . . . . . . . . . . . . . . . . . . . . . . .64

Pneumonia . . . . . . . . . . . . . . . . . . . . . . . . . . . . . . . . . . . . . . . . . . . 64

Poison Oak/Ivy Treatment . . . . . . . . . . . . . . . . . . . . . . . . . 65

Post Dermabrasion and Microdermabrasion . . . . . . . . . . . . . . 65

Post Peeling . . . . . . . . . . . . . . . . . . . . . . . . . . . . . . . . . . . . . . . . 66

Post Waxing or Hair Removal . . . . . . . . . . . . . . . . . . . . . . . . . 66

Radiation Burns . . . . . . . . . . . . . . . . . . . . . . . . . . . . . . . . . . . . . 67

Rashes. . . . . . . . . . . . . . . . . . . . . . . . . . . . . . . . . . . . . . . . . . . . . . . 67

Retro Viral Infection . . . . . . . . . . . . . . . . . . . . . . . . . . . . . . . . . 68

Scars . . . . . . . . . . . . . . . . . . . . . . . . . . . . . . . . . . . . . . . . . . . . . . . . 68

Shaving (Especially Sensitive Areas)/Razor Burn . . . . . . . . . 68

Shingles. . . . . . . . . . . . . . . . . . . . . . . . . . . . . . . . . . . . . . . . . . . . . . 69

Sinus Infections . . . . . . . . . . . . . . . . . . . . . . . . . . . . . . . . . . . . . . 69

Sore Throat . . . . . . . . . . . . . . . . . . . . . . . . . . . . . . . . . . . . . . . . . . 69

Stinky Feet . . . . . . . . . . . . . . . . . . . . . . . . . . . . . . . . . . . . . . . . . . 70

Sunburn . . . . . . . . . . . . . . . . . . . . . . . . . . . . . . . . . . . . . . . . . . . . . 70

Tattoo or Post Tattoo Removal. . . . . . . . . . . . . . . . . . . . . . . . . 71

Tooth Decay. . . . . . . . . . . . . . . . . . . . . . . . . . . . . . . . . . . . . . . . . . 72

Toenail Fungus. . . . . . . . . . . . . . . . . . . . . . . . . . . . . . . . . . . . . . . 73

Tonsillitis. . . . . . . . . . . . . . . . . . . . . . . . . . . . . . . . . . . . . . . . . . . . 73

Toys (Disinfection). . . . . . . . . . . . . . . . . . . . . . . . . . . . . . . . . . . . 74

Thrush . . . . . . . . . . . . . . . . . . . . . . . . . . . . . . . . . . . . . . . . . . . . . . . 74

Tuberculosis (TB). . . . . . . . . . . . . . . . . . . . . . . . . . . . . . . . . . . . . 74

Ulcers . . . . . . . . . . . . . . . . . . . . . . . . . . . . . . . . . . . . . . . . . . . . . . . 75

Upper Respiratory Tract Infections . . . . . . . . . . . . . . . . . . . . . 76

Urinary Tract Infections . . . . . . . . . . . . . . . . . . . . . . . . . . . . . . . 77

Vaginal Odor . . . . . . . . . . . . . . . . . . . . . . . . . . . . . . . . . . . . . . . . . 77

Vaginal Yeast Infection . . . . . . . . . . . . . . . . . . . . . . . . . . . . . . . . 78

Warts. . . . . . . . . . . . . . . . . . . . . . . . . . . . . . . . . . . . . . . . . . . . . . . . . 78

Water Purification. . . . . . . . . . . . . . . . . . . . . . . . . . . . . . . . . . . . . 78

References. . . . . . . . . . . . . . . . . . . . . . . . . . . . . . . . . . . . . . . . . . . . 81

## ABDOMINAL PAIN & DIARRHEA

Silver used at low levels in many case studies has shown that it can help reduce abdominal pain and discomfort quickly, especially when it is used as soon as possible at the onset of the symptoms. My suggestion is that you try drinking one ounce of a 10 ppm Nano silver product at the onset of the symptoms and then use two teaspoons, three times daily. In many cases the abdominal pain can be reduced within the first hour, and the diarrhea may be eliminated within the first day.

Some types of food poisoning can take more than one day to get rid of, especially if you have waited days to start using the silver and the bacteria has had a chance to build up in the system. But I have found that if you use the silver as soon as you feel the symptoms or sickness coming on, most types of stomach pain (abdominal pain) can go away within 10-30 minutes or so, and for most people the silver usually has a great soothing effect on the stomach. In my whole life I have only seen a few cases where people said that the silver actually caused the upset stomach. If that is the case stop using it and try something else.

## ACNE

The 24 ppm silver gel is a very valuable tool in the fight against acne. First, if it is necessary to pop a zit, the application of the gel can help keep the damaged skin from becoming infected. It can also help reduce the inflammation of the agitated skin (help it keep from swelling up big). The silver gel can also help the zit to heal about twice as fast as normal. If you pop a zit, liberally apply the gel to the area in and around the zit and let it soak in. For daily use to help reduce acne, wash the face or affected area first with water or the 10 ppm Nano silver liquid. Then, apply a liberal amount of the 24 ppm silver gel to your hands, rub your hands together and then apply to the face or other acne prone area. Gently rub the gel onto the face or affected area and then let it soak in. The silver gel is more effective in helping eliminate bacterial acne than it is against hormonal acne. Expect to see significant results within the first week or two. In one study completed in Japan, women put the 24 ppm gel on their face twice a day, morning and night, daily for two months. At the end of two months, the women showed an average of a 17% reduction in facial blemish. The 10 ppm liquid is also used by many people as a facial toner.

## AIDS

See HIV.

## ALLERGIES

Using the 10 ppm Nano silver liquid will not cure allergies, but the anti-inflammatory effect seems to help reduce the symptoms very significantly. You may want to take up to two teaspoons three times daily. Usually you will find a significant reduction in symptoms within hours to a day. Using the 10 ppm Nano silver liquid up in the nose seems to help dry the flow of a runny nose within a few minutes. Empty a nasal sprayer, refill with the 10 ppm Nano silver liquid and use as needed: a few times daily is usually enough.

## ANIMAL USES

Animal treatments are much the same as those described for humans. Both the Nano silver gel and the liquid have been shown to be nontoxic to animals in both ingested and injected studies. One advantage of using the Nano silver gel for the wounds of animals like horses etc., is that flies and some other biting bugs for some reason do not seem to like the taste of the 24 ppm Nano silver gel and so they avoid landing on the wound treatment areas reducing the possible spread of infection.

## ANTIBIOTIC USE

The use of Nano silver liquids with antibiotics can be a very good one-two punch against problem diseases and infection. I do not usually condone the use of antibiotics unless they are really needed and the problem pathogen is neither a yeast nor virus, over which antibiotics have little effect. Two studies(6,14) have shown that the use of liquid silver with antibiotics has made the antibiotics as much as 10–1000 times more effective. The silver can also eliminate resistant bacteria that the antibiotics usually cannot. So if you need to use antibiotics for some reason, it would probably go very well for you to use some 10 ppm Nano silver at a level of 2 teaspoons three times daily, while taking the antibiotics. I have seen no negative interaction between the use of silver and the antibiotics to date. One published study showed that in 96 tests using 19 different antibiotics and seven different pathogens, using the Nano silver liquid with the antibiotics had either additive or synergistic value in all but two.[6]

# ASTHMA

One of the most interesting reports coming from people using the Nano silver may be the effect it seems to have on asthma. Several people have reported that the silver solution taken orally can reduce the number and also the severity of asthma attacks. One individual reported that he has suffered from asthma since he was five years old and had to use Broncho-dilators up to six times a day. He stated that he started taking the Nano silver 10 ppm for a deep chest cough and was surprised when after about 10 days his asthma attacks completely ceased. He reported that he was taking two teaspoons of the 10 ppm silver Nano solution every three to four hours during the day when the attacks stopped. He then stopped taking the solution to see if it was really the silver that helped the asthma. The asthma attacks again came back after about three days. He then restarted taking the Nano silver solution and again the asthma symptoms reduced. After taking the initial dose for about a month, he cut his use to two teaspoons in the morning and two at night. He reported that new dosage seemed to be sufficient help prevent the recurrence of asthma attacks. It has been suggested by a number of researchers that the Nano silver has important anti-inflammatory properties. This may explain the benefit of the silver solution in the treatment of asthma symptoms, which is caused by the inflammation of the bronchial tubes.

# ATHLETE'S FOOT

Athlete's foot can be a big problem for many people, especially those that regularly work out in a public gym. It can cause both a nasty odor and an itching and burning sensation on the feet. In most light cases, just applying the 24 ppm Nano silver gel generously to the affected areas morning, noon, and night, is sufficient to eliminate the problem.

For almost immediate relief of itching, the gel can be applied as often as needed. The Nano silver gel has the ability to both kill the nasty odor causing microbes and also soothe the itch and burn of the skin.

In tough cases I suggest that you purchase some hydrogen peroxide from your local drug store and mix it half and half with the 10 ppm Nano silver liquid product. Put the Nano silver/ hydrogen peroxide mix product in a small spray bottle and spray the affected area of the feet three times daily. Once the feet are sprayed, let it dry and then apply the Nano silver gel over the top of the dried silver/peroxide mix.

In most cases, even the most stubborn strains of athlete's food cannot survive this protocol. In severe cases it can take up to a couple of weeks to get rid of the problem, but most people will find at least some relief very quickly.

# BEDSORES

Bedsores are a type of skin ulcer called a pressure ulcer. They usually happen to elderly people who stay in one position too long, like sitting in a wheelchair or lying in a bed. The 24 ppm gel is very useful in helping to close or heal a bedsore. Simply apply a generous amount of the 24 ppm Nano silver gel to the affected area twice daily, and keep covered. Good things will usually start happening within just a few days as the inflammation around the wound subsides and healing begins. There are a lot of factors in how long it will take to help resolve the wound, like how big it was when treatment was started and also the condition of the patient.

# BIRD FLU

Bird flu is caused by a deadly virus. There are many different strains of bird flu. They are some of the most deadly types of influenza that exists. It has been stated that the 1918 flu that reportedly killed 25-50 million people worldwide was a bird flu. The new strains that are now being reported and are killing a few people are said to be even more deadly than the 1918 strain, and could go pandemic at any time. The real problem with bird flu is that people can have the disease and be able to spread it to other people around them for as long as 10 days before they show any symptoms or even know that they have the disease. There are a number of studies where the engineered silver Nano-particles were put up against a number of different strains of bird flu. In the test tube, the Silver Nano particles were able to kill or neutralize each and every strain tested so far.

There was also completed an animal model published report[9] where it was found that using the Nano silver liquid every day for a week before being infected, saved over half the animals from being killed by the deadly bird flu. In other words, using a little bit of the 10 ppm Nano silver product twice a day as an immune support supplement helped 100% more of the animals survive the deadly disease. The survival rate increased from 30% to 60% with just seven days of daily usage before they were infected. The other good news is that a 10 ppm product is safe enough to use every day.

When it comes to treating the flu, it is generally much easier to help prevent it by daily use of the silver than it is to cure it once you have it. The difference is that once the virus has had time to build up in your system, it takes a while for the silver to help your body to eliminate it. The reason for this is that a virus replicates inside your cells and the Nano silver will not enter your cells to get to the virus. So it can only eliminate the virus once the virus ruptures or kills the cells. The Nano silver can then hunt down the new virus and neutralize them before they can infect a new cell. Usually using the silver daily would help a sick person get over a case of the flu in about half the normal time. I would suggest using the silver at about two teaspoons, used three times daily. General prevention would be at one teaspoon three times daily. You can double up on the use of the 10 ppm liquid for protection if people around you start showing signs of coming down with the flu.

## BLACK MOLD

Black mold is a nasty form of mold which typically grows in damp areas and can infect the lungs of people living in the area. The spore that comes from the mold can actually grow in the lungs, causing respiratory infections. To eliminate mold on hard surfaces, just spray the 10 ppm Nano silver directly on the mold. The 10 ppm will kill mold in about 10–15 minutes.[26] Simply spray it on the surface leave it for the 10–15 minutes and then wipe it off. Do not spray on porous areas, the silver can dry in the little holes and then discolor the item. Any hard or quality painted, water resistant surface is OK. It also seems that once you spray an area, even after you wipe it off, enough silver stays behind to help keep the mold from growing back for months and possibly even much longer.

To help treat a lung infection, put the 10 ppm Nano silver in a nebulizer and breath in about 5-10 ml. two to three times daily. By using a nebulizer you can get full strength product directly on the mold in the lungs, it should help clear the lungs in just a few days to a week. One doctor I know found big mushrooms of black mold growing inside a wall near the window well, it was making the whole family sick. He removed the sheetrock, treated the areas to kill the mold, and then used a nebulizer to help clear it from the lungs of his family members. He reported that it worked really well.

## BODY ODOR

Body odor can be caused by bacteria. To reduce body odor, try applying the 24 ppm Nano silver gel liberally to the area of the body that smells. The gel will help eliminate the odor within 10-15 minutes. Massage therapists can benefit by the use of the gel on patients that smell. Not only will the gel help make their skin incredibly soft in minutes, but it will help kill the odor causing bacteria, thus making the job much easier for the massage therapist. This odor reduction action will also be much appreciated by ladies that wear sandals without socks in the hot summer and also by parents who have teenage boys or girls with stinky feet. The odor killing action of the gel is also used a lot by bow hunters who are working to eliminate body odor, so animals cannot smell them while in the field.

## BRONCHITIS

I suggest you take two teaspoons of the 10 ppm Nano Silver liquid three times daily. Most people report feeling signs of recovery in about two days and report full recovery in less than a week. Many people are finding accelerated relief using the Nano silver liquid in a nebulizer, where they inhale (one teaspoon/5 ml) the cold mist three times a day until the condition is resolved. The benefit of the nebulizer is that it puts full-strength product directly on the pathogen in the lungs.

## BUG BITES/SPIDER BITES

The Nano silver product seems to be very helpful when it comes to bug bites. The bite of a mosquito can cause an itching reaction. By just applying the 24 ppm Nano silver gel to the effected skin, the gel can usu-ally make the itch go away within just a few minutes (10–15 minutes). I have done the same thing with a wasp sting and found the same kind of relief within a few minutes. I had a nice woman call me from Hawaii and report that she had been bitten by a large blue centipede. She said that it was a lot like being stung by a wasp. She stated that she had poured some of the 10 ppm liquid product onto a cotton ball and had held it on the bite. She reported that within 10–15 minutes, the pain was gone and that the swelling had subsided.

Spider bites can be a very big problem. They get infected easily and can lead to big problems, including amputation and even death. One mil-itary man I have worked with had a son that was bitten by a spider. The son did not treat the bite with the silver. By the second day the bite area on his hand had swollen to almost twice its normal size. The military man, who also happens to be a doctor, lanced the infected part of the bite and applied the silver onto the wound. He told me that by the next morning most of the swelling had subsided and the bite was looking much better.

I have had many people report similar stories to me with similar re-sults. I have also seen the bulls eye spider bite pustules go away in as little as two to three days. I believe that the Nano silver products have the ability to neutralize toxins associated with the bite. The usual protocol for treating a spider bite is to first lance the pustule, wash it out with the liquid Nano silver, put the gel into the hole as the healing agent, and then cover the bite with a bandage. The pronounced anti-inflammatory action of the gel usually helps reduce the size of the bite as well as make the bite feel better. Healing occurs rapidly; usually within only a few days. For any serious bug or spider bite, make sure you see your doctor or health care provider.

## BURNS & CUTS

If you have a cut, you can wash it out or clean it with the 10 ppm Nano silver product. This will not only help clean the wound but it will also start the disinfection process (kill the germs). Once the cut has been cleaned, you can apply the 24 ppm silver gel directly onto the burn or cut in a generous manner. I would suggest you use it up to 3 times/day depending on severity of the wound and how often the bandages need changing. Covering the wound with a sterile bandage will help keep the wound moist and help reduce the amount of scaring that occurs. If the wound is painful to the touch, like a burn, the silver gel can be placed directly on the bandage and then placed on the wound.

Most people report that burns and cuts are healing very rapidly, some almost twice as fast. In one published case study,[10] an 88 year old woman with massive third degree burns down the inside of both legs was treated with the Nano silver gel. The 24 ppm gel was applied once daily, when the bandages were changed out. The report shows that the Nano silver was able to help regrow the skin on the legs in 65days.

Once a person has been burned, it is important to apply the gel rapidly. This will do several things. One, it will have a direct cooling effect which will stop the burn from continuing to burn and doing more damage to the skin and tissue. Secondly, it will start the anti-inflammatory response and that will help reduce the pain associated with the burn.

A sunburn is a type of radiation burn that can effect almost everyone at some time in their lives. A sunburn is very much like the burns that cancer patients can get from radiation therapy. One cancer clinic I know has used 24 ppm Nano silver gel to help treat the burns after radiation treatment. The doctor told me that when the patients use the gel they reported that the silver gel product caused an instantaneous cooling effect on the burns and that the burns were healing in about half the normal time, with much reduced pain. The Nano Silver gel seems to work well with all three types of burns, including heat, radiation and also chemical burns. The Nano silver is also being reported to help reduce the scaring associated with the burns. It sometimes helps to apply the gel to the burn area two to three times within the first few hours of being burned. It is important to use the gel as soon as possible (ASAP) in order to minimize the continuation of the burning effect on the skin.

# CANCERS

Cancers can be difficult, torturous, and deadly. I do not think there are any easy answers to treating it once you have it. That being said, I think that silver could play a big role in helping to keep people from getting cancer and can also play a serious role in helping people who develop cancer and are in treatment.

First on the list is that it has been reported that about 60% of cancer types have been linked to some sort of pathogen, like HPV and cervical cancer for example (for treatment protocols see HPV). So the ability of Nano silver to kill a broad spectrum of pathogens, with daily use, may help eliminate the development of many types of cancer.

Secondly, it is possible that silver could uncloak tumor cancer cells so that the body's immune system can recognize that the cells are not functioning properly and could kill them. It has been reported that the body's immune system kills cancer cells in its normal function and that having a healthy immune system can help keep people from developing cancer. For cancer to take over in a body, the cancerous cells must remain hidden from the body's immune system.

In a very interesting test case, a scientist I know had a dog with a tumor on his neck. The tumor was very large and was killing the dog. In an attempt to save his beloved dog, the scientist tried injecting the 10 ppm Nano silver into the tumor of the dog with a syringe. He injected the dog's tumor once a day, in a different place on three consecutive days. He then reported a very interesting effect. He reported that the skin developed a small hole or abscess, where the silver had been injected and that the tumor in that spot was melting away and running out the hole. He said the liquid draining from the tumor resembled green tea and that the drainage was occurring at each of the three injection sites and that the tumor was visibly shrinking at each of the sites. His theory is that the silver was somehow effecting the cancers ability to hide (possibly effecting a protein) and that the immune system had recognized that the cancer at the injection site was there, and that the body's own immune system was killing those infected cells. What he may have discovered is a possible treatment for at least some types of cancerous tumors. I realize that this is very preliminary data. But, in order to develop protocols and test the theory, the idea has to be put forth so that smarter and more knowledgeable doctors can add more data and test the theory to see if it is of value.

The third area entails the treatment (closing) of skin cancer lesions. I have had numerous reports where the Nano silver has helped to close or heal open skin cancer sores. By applying the gel directly on the open skin sore three times daily, people are reporting visual healing is occurring quickly and that results of the 24 ppm Nano silver gel helping to heal the wound can be seen in as little as a week.

The fourth area of impact silver can have on cancer has more to do with treatment than prevention. Nano silver is a great healing agent, and it is also anti-inflammatory and antimicrobial. As such, it can play a major role in helping treat the side effects of cancer treatments. One cancer treatment center in California has treated thousands of patients with radiation to kill cancer cells. As a side effect of the treatment, the radiation therapy burns the skin of the patient, causing both pain and discomfort. One of the cancer doctors reported to me that all of his patients loved using the 24 ppm Nano silver gel. He said that the silver gel caused an almost instantaneous cooling and soothing effect on the radiation burned areas of skin. He also said that the radiation burns were healing in about half the normal time, which was reported as a fantastic result. The patients simply apply the gel in a generous manner to the burned area as needed for comfort, but at least three times daily.

Another area of possible treatment use is to use the silver liquid as a supplement at least three times daily. Many cancer treatment protocols use poisons like chemo therapy to kill cancer cells. The hope is that the chemo treatment will kill more cancer cells than healthy cells, but that does not always happen. One of the losers in the battle is usually the body's white blood cells, which can also be killed by the chemo, leaving the body unprotected from other pathogenic invaders. The silver, used as a supplement, can help boost or replace the white blood cells in the bloodstream, to help keep the patient who is being treated for cancer, from getting sick and possibly dying from another pathogenic invader or sickness. As an idea for use, and if it were me receiving cancer treatment, I would drink about two ounces daily TID (split into taking 4 teaspoons in the morning, at noon and then again at night). I believe that by this use, the Nano silver 10 ppm can help function as a type of second immune system, or first line of defense, to help back up the function of your normal immune system and help protect the sick person undergoing treatment.

The last area of cancer treatment with 10 ppm Nano silver is probably one of the most interesting. I have yet to really understand it, but lately I have been getting numerous reports of people taking mega doses of the

Nano silver 10 ppm over relatively short periods of time and having some very interesting results.

One case reported was a women in Hawaii with a very advanced leukemia type of cancer. Her brother had died from the same type of cancer. One of her family members had her using about 8 ounces daily of the Nano silver liquid in divided doses (that is a little more than 2.5 ounces three times daily). Surprisingly with the daily doses she started to feel better and better. About 30 days later she went back to the doctor and found that she tested negative for the cancer, it was all gone. There is a strong possibility that the mega doses of the silver boosted her immune system, which then was able to eliminate the cancer from her body. I have also received a number of other cancer reports where mega dosing for 30 to 60 days has showed also very positive results.

## CANKERS & OTHER MOUTH SORES

Take approximately 1 tablespoon of liquid product into mouth. Hold in mouth on affected area for at least 5-6 minutes, or as long as you can if five minutes is too much. Repeat 2-3 times daily or more if needed. Noticeable improvements are being reported by the next day on almost all cankers and most other mouth sores. Some people report that pain may start to subside within as little as an hour. I had one of my scouts tell me that he could not eat. When a scout will not eat, you know that something is very wrong, because they are eating machines. When I asked him what was wrong he told me that he had about five canker sores in his mouth and that it was just too painful to eat. I talked to his parents and they agreed to try the silver. The scout placed the product in his mouth using the instructions as stated above, and told me that all the pain was gone by the next day, just as I thought it would be.

## CHICKEN POX

Chicken Pox are a virus that causes spots (almost like a zit) to form, sometimes all over the body. It can be a light case with just a few red spots or there can be hundreds. The 24 ppm Nano silver gel works well to help take the burn and itch out of the spots. Putting the gel on the sores will also help keep them from becoming infected and also help them to go away faster. Simply rub a generous amount of the gel on each of the spots, the itch should subside in about 10-30 minutes. The gel will also help heal the spots in about half the normal time. Taking two teaspoons of the 10 ppm liquid three times daily, can also help reduce the symptoms and the sick down time.

## COLD SORES

Saturate a cotton ball with the silver solution, apply to lip 2-3 times per day. Using the product more than three times a day can help a lot with the swelling and generally ugly look of a cold sore. Keep the wet cotton ball in direct contact with the cold sore for at least 5 minutes and as long as 30 minutes. Most people report that when applied in this manner, and if applied before the cold sore actually breaks into a blister (when you feel that first itch), a blister may never appear. If the blister has already appeared or even if it has already broken, the silver product can reduce the healing time greatly. Noticeable improvements have been made in 1-3 days. The earlier it is applied, the better it seems to work. It seems to be able to not only reduce the swelling, but also to kill or neutralize the virus that causes the cold sore, and also help heal the wound in just a few days.

I seem to get cold sores when I sunburn my lips. Before the silver was available to me, I could suffer from a cold sore for as many as 3-4 weeks. Every morning when I took a shower it would just seem to get bigger. Now by using the silver as stated above, even if a blister has broken out, the cold sore is scabbed over by the next day and is gone usually in just three to four days.

## COMMON COLDS

The Nano silver liquid appears to be more effective as a prophylactic (preventative) than as a cure for the common cold. For prevention, take one teaspoon two to three times daily. If used after the onset of a cold, the Nano silver product usually helps to cut recuperation time in half. To help speed recuperation time, take two teaspoons three times daily.

## DANDRUFF

After showering and washing the hair, dry off and then massage a small amount of the 10 ppm liquid into the scalp. This will help the skin to become much healthier, and help to eliminate problems that can cause the skin to dry and fall off (dandruff). It can also help to eliminate the itch associated with scalp irritations. For whatever reason this scalp treatment also seems to give the hair great body, without making it look greasy. One 80+ year old man also kept reporting to me that massaging the scalp with the 10 ppm Nano liquid was causing new hair growth to occur on previously balding areas of his head. His thought was that the liquid Nano silver was killing some pathogen that was inhibiting the natural hair growth. I have seen no proof that what he said was true, but I do believe that massaging the scalp with the Nano silver can help with scalp problem in a big way.

A number of people I know also use the 24 ppm Nano silver gel as a hair gel, giving them a double protection against scalp problems. The silver gel seems to function much the same as most of the regular hair gels, but with the added value of being both antimicrobial and a natural healing agent.

## DENTAL APPLICATIONS

There are probably hundreds of dental applications for the use of both the Nano silver gel and liquid. For example, the liquid 10 ppm Nano silver is being used as a mouthwash to kill both odor causing bacteria and also to kill tooth decay causing bacteria. The liquid is also being used as a mouthwash after oral surgery to help minimize the potential of post-op infections. The liquid can also be used to hydrate the bone cement used after root canals. The Nano liquid silver can make the bone cement antibacterial, which can help eliminate the potential of further tooth decay from inside the tooth. The liquid silver can also be used in a water dental pick after scaling, which pressure sprays the liquid up under the gum line to help kill the bacteria and to help start to shrink the perio pockets.

The 24 ppm Nano silver gel also has numerous applications for use in the dental arena. I am aware of a number of new patents that have been filed covering some of these uses. The gel can be used after the removal of wisdom teeth. One DMD told me that he has performed more than 10,000 oral surgeries using the gel as part of the post op protocols. He told me that after he removes a tooth he washes out the hole (can use the liquid 10 ppm), and then he puts a layer of gel in the bottom. He then puts in a thin collagen membrane, and then another layer of gel. He then sows the skin flap closing the wound. He reported that his patients are reporting no pain by days 2-3, no squirrel cheek inflammation, and heal rates of about half the normal time. He also told me that he had had only about three secondary infections out of the first 300 cases, and he said those were mostly associated with the ripping open of his dental work in bar fights (hockey season). He said that he always places gel in the wound before sewing any skin flap closed.

Another dentist told me that he has been putting the gel into tooth trays and having his patients leave them in their mouths for several hours. He said that using the gel in the tooth tray has helped eliminate gingivitis in as little as 1-3 days.

Numerous dentists have also had their patients use the 24 ppm Nano silver gel as a tooth gel, like a toothpaste. The gel has no color, smell, or toxicity if swallowed, and has been shown to immensely help reduce redness and swelling of the gums. I have used it for years and it still surprises me that when I wake up in the morning, after having brushed my teeth with the gel at night, my mouth still feels squeaky clean like no bad bacteria could grow in it.

I also know that several new dental tooth gels have already been engineered for use in the dental industry and will soon be available on the market. Those new dental gel products will contain the 24 ppm Nano silver as a main ingredient with xylitol and peppermint oil, all three being natural bacteria killers. I believe that those new tooth gel products can and will have a significant positive impact on dental health worldwide, killing bacteria and helping to heal the gums. I believe that the new tooth gel will not foam in the mouth but will go on smooth and make the teeth and gums feel really smooth for hours and hours.

# DIABETIC NEUROPATHY (SORES)

Because of impaired circulation, it is common for people with diabetes to have cuts and scratches heal very slowly, and many times they get worse and worse until finally doctors amputate the part (usually a toe or finger). To avoid this, wash out the wound with the 10 ppm liquid and then cover the entire wound with the 24 ppm Nano silver gel, and then cover the wound with a nonstick bandage. Repeat this protocol daily. You need a nonstick bandage because when you change out the bandage you do not want to rip out the newly formed skin or tissue.

Using the gel on the diabetic cuts etc., has had an amazing effect. One man had had an open diabetic wound on his back the size of an apple. He said it had been unable to heal for many years. Using the gel daily in the wound helped close it within five months. I have also seen a case where an amputation was scheduled to cut off a man's toes, but by using the 24 ppm Nano silver gel the wound was healed and the amputation was avoided completely. Most of the dime-sized wounds heal within 3-5 weeks, which is really slow for a normal person but amazingly fast for a diabetic. Using the gel appears to not only shorten healing times, but it also helps to reduce pain in the extremities. The gel will also help kill the odor causing bacteria that may be on the feet. Daily use may help eliminate potential wounds in areas prone to having diabetic ulcer problems.

## DIAPER AND OTHER RASHES

Most diaper rashes are caused by either a bacteria or a yeast. Either way it does not matter, the Nano silver will kill both. For diaper rash, spray affected area with 10ppm Nano silver liquid at each change of diaper as you clean the area. Once the area is clean, cover the entire effected area with a thin layer of the 24 ppm Nano silver gel, then replace the diaper with a new one. Repeat at least three times per day. Most people find that the gel will have a great soothing effect on the pain and redness associated with the diaper rash, which can occur within as little as 20-30 minutes. Many people have been reporting a very noticeable change for the better by the next morning.

Most diaper rashes are gone in just 1–3 days depending on the severity of the problem and when the product is first used. I have only seen a few cases that did not respond very quickly to the use of the silver gel, and I think that those cases were caused by some sort of allergic reaction instead of a pathogen (problem bacteria etc.). If this happens I suggest you discontinue use and seek the help of a good pediatrician (children's doctor).

# DISINFECTION OF CUTTING BOARDS

There are many bacterial infections that come through the food we eat. Bacteria like E. coli and also Salmonella to name just a few. Many people think that these poisonous bacteria are just associated with meats, especially fish. This is not true. Many food poisons come from the contamination of fresh vegetables used in salads or just eaten raw. The silver Nano particles have been shown to be extremely effective at killing these pathogens (harmful bacteria).

Nano silver has easily killed every form of food poisoning bacteria that I have ever seen. Spray foods and cooking surfaces before and after preparing meals. Do not use the silver on surfaces that are porous (have small micro-sized holes in it). If you do, the silver will get down in the holes and, when dry, can discolor light colored objects. Cutting boards and other hard non-porous surfaces are no problem at all. Spray the object, wait 10 minutes for the silver to kill the bacteria, and then wipe clean with a paper towel.

# EAR ACHES BOTH INTERNAL AND EXTERNAL

Most ear infections are caused by a Streptococcus pneumonia and H. influenzas bacteria. I have seen it proven that a 10 ppm liquid product can easily kill both of these bacteria. To treat the ear infection, just lay the person or child down on bed or soft couch with affected ear facing up. Place 5-7 drops of the silver solution in the infected ear. Remain in this laying down position for at least 10 minutes and it is better if the person stays laying down with the ear up for as long as 30 minutes. Repeat 2-3 times daily. Most people are reporting good results in as little as 12-24 hours. This use is very important, because 7 out of 10 kids suffer from ear infections by the age of three years old.

I had ear aches as a child and it is a very painful experience. I have been asked a number of times if kids who have tubes in their ears can use the silver. These kids usually have tubes because they have suffered with many middle ear infections (Otitis Media). The tubes are placed in the ear to both release the pressure inside the ear, which helps reduce the pain, and also to provide a drain for the bacteria laden puss that comes from the infection. The tubes actually make it easier for the silver to get to the problem middle-ear bacteria to kill it. So in direct answer to the question, I have never seen any problem with kids with tubes in their ears using the silver liquid to help combat the problem bacteria. We have seen very good results against both otitis externa and otitis media (both internal and external ear infections).

A few people want to argue about how the silver can get into the middle ear to kill the bacteria if no tube is present and the ear drum has not ruptured. The point is that the kids don't really care, just try it once for yourself and you will see how well it works. The good news for doctors who work in clinics doing humanitarian work, is that by using the Nano silver product in this protocol, a doctor my help more than a hundred kids with ear infections with just one 8 ounce bottle. The protocol also works really well for dogs, although it is difficult to get them to settle down long enough to give the silver a chance to work. One vet I talked to sedates the dogs first and then uses the silver in their ears. He reported great success.

## EBOLA

EBOLA is a deadly virus that has been around for more than a decade, but recently has shown signs of becoming pandemic, meaning that it may have been able to evolve into a disease that may spread easily and rapidly around the world. It is a disease that is spread by contact with body fluids, like blood, urine, sperm, or spit, but rumor has it that it may have mutated to where it can move by air, breathed out by an infected person. I have seen no proof of that, but I do believe that it has spread far beyond what has been reported. One report that I read said that whole villages were quarantined, more than a million people in total. The bad news is that it has been killing more than half the people that get infected with it.

The virus infects the blood and can destroy or rupture very small blood vessels. Since the silver travels the same routes in the blood and can come in direct contact with the virus just by drinking some, I have theorized that chances were very good that the Nano silver would have a very positive effect against the virus. Recent human tests are proving that theory to be correct. A group of 89 unpublished case studies in Africa have showed that a 10 ppm Nano silver has been able help infected people recover in just days.

One Nigerian scientist has been using the 10 ppm orally (drinking it) at level of about 4 tablespoons (two ounces) taken three times daily, the patients have recovered in about 5 days. A report from a very knowledgeable Egyptian doctor expanded the protocols to include not only oral ingestion of approximately 1 table spoon taken every six hours before food, but also breathing in 8 ml. (a little more than one teaspoon) twice daily of the 10 ppm Nano silver in a nebulizer. By taking it in through both the mouth and the lungs he reported that he was also achieving serious recovery within just a few days.

## ECZEMA

Eczema can be a very itchy and scaly problem for many people. It makes them very self-conscious around other people. The Nano silver gel seems to do amazing things for eczema. The liquid will also work in helping the condition, it is just not as easy to use. The gel can be used to both eliminate the itch and also to heal the affected areas. A neighbor of mine had a two-year-old boy who had eczema covering the entire top of his head. It was scaly with scabs, and it would bleed when he scratched at the scabs. His mom asked if she could try the silver and I gave it to her. She covered the affected area with the Nano silver a number of times a day. Within a month, the child's head was clear and clean, with no evidence of any remaining eczema. I have also received other reports that were very similar in nature. I would suggest a protocol of covering the affected area with the 24 ppm gel at least three to four times daily. I would expect to see improvement within the first week, and resolution of the case within the first month or sooner for a mild or moderate case. A severe case may take longer. When used for the itch or burn associated with the condition, I would anticipate that applying the gel would help soothe or get rid of the itch within 15–30 minutes.

## EMERGENCY STORAGE

Because Nano silver products are very stable, it is a very good idea to add some cases of both the liquid and the gel products into any emergency storage preparations. Problems can happen at any time and both natural disasters and manmade problems can limit your ability to get food, water, or any medicine at all. Hurricane Katrina showed that it can take up to weeks and weeks for the government to get aid into areas devastated by a natural disaster. The most difficult thing about a disaster might be the pain of watching loved ones die from simple problems that could have easily been solved with the help of Nano silver products.

Stability testing on the 10 ppm Nano silver liquid shows that in official tests, there was no degeneration of the product over a period of seven years and one month. Unofficial reports show that the Nano silver liquid is still very effective even after 12 years of sitting in a PETE, food grade, plastic bottle. A university study found that glass may not be a good long term storage container for silver liquids.[18] The study found that glass could negatively affect the silver and that it could fall out of solution and become of little use. The 24 ppm Nano silver gel has been shown to be very effective even after 5 years, the limiting factor in the gel is not the Nano silver, but that the gelling agents start to break down after a number of years. The Nano silver gel does not go bad, it just becomes a little less effective over the long term.

# EYE INFECTIONS

The US EPA has reported that silver is neither an eye nor skin irritant. [3] Silver nitrate has also been used in the eyes of newborn babies for over a hundred years because of its ability to combat eye infections. The Nano silver liquids can be very effective in helping to combat eye infections, even pink eye. In two reported human case studies in Africa, the doctors reported cases of eye infections. The doctors treated the eye infections by putting just a few drops of the 10 ppm Nano silver product right in the infected eye. They reported that the eye infections were fully recovered in an average of just one day. I have used the product for my own children for pink eye. I found that by putting about two-three drops of product into the corner of the eye and by having them blink the eye, so that the silver made it into the inside of the eye lid, then holding the eye closed for about five minutes to give the silver time to work, three times a day, that the pink eye was showing good signs of recovery by the very next day and was completely gone by the end of the third day.

By following this protocol, most regular eye infections are cleared very rapidly, usually within the first day or two. I also know a number of people who have sprayed the silver liquid into tired or painful eyes. The anti-inflammatory nature of the silver seems to help soothe the condition very rapidly. If the eyes are really sore the placement of the silver liquid in the eyes can cause a slight stinging sensation, the effect will usually go away quickly and will be replaced by the wonderful soothing sensation within a very few minutes.

## EYE (TIRED EYES)

I have found that spraying the 10 ppm Nano silver in my eyes can help relieve tired eye syndrome, meaning the burning and itch of tired and strained eyes. To use simply spray or drip a few drops of the 10 ppm liquid directly into the eyes. Once the silver is in the eyes, close them for 5-10 minutes. By closing the eyes with the silver in them, it will give the silver time to work. I believe it will not only kill any bacteria, etc. in the eyes, but the anti-inflammatory nature of the silver will help soothe the eyes and make them feel better. The EPA red document on silver states that silver is neither an eye nor skin irritant.[3] As stated above, if the eyes are really sore the placement of the silver liquid in the eyes can cause a slight stinging sensation, the effect will usually go away quickly and will be replaced by the wonderful soothing sensation within a very few minutes.

## FACIALS

Facials can be enhanced in a major way, with the addition of silver products. The liquid is great as an antimicrobial wash and also facial toner. The 24 ppm gel will make the skin feel incredibly soft in about two minutes. It will also provide an antimicrobial layer of protection on the skin that will last for about four hours. To use, simply apply the gel to the face and gently massage into the skin. The Nano silver gel will make the skin feel soft in about 2 minutes. In a non-published Japanese study, a woman who used the 24 ppm Nano silver gel morning and night, showed a 17% reduction in facial blemish in just two months of daily use. I believe that over time, the Nano silver gel helped replace small scar tissue blemishes with new clean skin.

# FLU

Take two teaspoons of the of the 10 ppm Nano silver liquid at least 2-3 times daily by mouth. An adult can safely drink six teaspoons a day, and when fighting a flu virus it may help to do so. Hold the solution in your mouth (gargle if possible) for three to five minutes before swallowing. Noticeable improvements have been reported in 1-3 days, especially if taken at onset of sickness. Slower success rates are reported if only taken after the bacteria or virus has become entrenched in the body. Remember the average flu can easily last 14 days with no treatment, so if the silver can help to get rid of it in just a day or two, it will have done its job well.

If someone in your family gets the flu, it is important to have the rest of the family use the Nano silver liquid daily, so that it may help boost their immune systems. This may help protect the rest of the family and help keep the sickness from spreading to other family members. Remember though, even if they do not show symptoms, many of the other family members may have already been infected with the flu virus. For this reason it is important to have the rest of the family use the 10 ppm liquid while someone in the family is sick.

When it comes to treating the flu, generally it is much easier to help prevent it by daily use of the silver than it is to cure it once you have it. The difference is that once the virus has had time to build up in your system, it takes a while for the silver to help your body to eliminate it. The reason for this is that a virus replicates inside your cells and the Nano silver will not enter your cells to get to the virus. So it can only eliminate the virus once the virus ruptures or kills the cell. The Nano silver can then help hunt down the new virus and neutralize them before they can infect a new cell.

# FOOD POISONING

Testing of the 10 ppm Nano silver products has proven their ability to kill numerous types of bacteria that may cause food poisoning. Those bacteria include; E. coli, Salmonella, Listeria, and Staphylococcus. To use, try drinking one ounce (six teaspoons) of a 10 ppm Nano silver liquid solution at onset of upset stomach or as soon as you can get some. Positive results have been reported in as little as 10 minutes, and as long as 3 hours. It is important to use the product as soon as possible when you start to feel sick, so that bacteria levels in the body can be minimized before they have time to build up in the body and spread into the blood stream.

It is also widely believed that the silver products can also help precipitate out many of the toxic proteins that can be released when some food poisoning bacteria are killed. This may help to explain why some cases of suspected food poisoning can be managed so quickly. As a follow up, drink two teaspoons of the 10 ppm Nano silver three times daily, until all the symptoms are resolved.

## FUNGAL / YEAST SKIN INFECTIONS

Many fungal skin infections are eliminated very quickly by the Nano silver products. To use, liberally spread the 24 ppm Nano silver gel over the affected area. The gel will usually help eliminate the burn or itch associated with the infection within 15-20 minutes, and will help eliminate the problem within a few days.

## FUNGUS INFECTIONS OF THE FEET:

Foot fungal infections can be difficult to treat, as many have become very resistant to products designed to kill or eliminate them. The silver gel can easily eliminate most of them. To use, wash the feet well with soap and water, dry and then rub a goodly amount of the 24 ppm Nano silver gel on the affected areas. Repeat three to four times daily.

For stubborn athletes foot fungus, I suggest a pretreatment of 10 ppm Nano silver liquid, mixed half and half with a 3% hydrogen peroxide solution (available from any drug store). After mixing the 10 ppm liquid with the hydrogen peroxide, place the mixed product in a spray bottle. After washing the feet, spray the silver/hydrogen peroxide mix on the affected area, let dry, then apply the 24 ppm Nano silver gel to the area. Repeat 2-4 times daily. This double-action attack seems to do very well, even against some stubborn strains. This process should also easily relieve the itching and help eliminate the possible stinky odor caused by the foot infection.

## GENERAL WELL-BEING

It is widely suspected that much of the time we feel run-down and tired, that what we actually have is a low-grade infection. If we do not take care of ourselves in those circumstances, the infection often blossoms and we become really sick. Take one teaspoon of the 10 ppm Nano silver liquid, two or three times daily, as a mineral supplement. Most people find that if they take a few teaspoons of the 10 ppm product each day, they rarely get sick. And the few times that people report getting sick when using the product daily, they report that the sickness is usually a very light case and seldom lasts longer than a day.

I know one older couple who reported that the husband got sick every fall and would continue to be sick until April or May. They called me to thank me because he was using the 10 ppm Nano silver liquid product daily and had made it an entire year without being sick. I use the product mostly daily and have for almost 17 years. Sometimes I forget and I may go a week or two without taking it. In the 17 years I have been taking the product I have only been sick twice, and that was mostly because I had been traveling by plane or boat and had been exposed to many sick people and I did not have enough silver with me at the time to help keep my immune system at a high level.

## GINGIVITIS

A lot of people suffer from Gingivitis. The 24 ppm Nano silver gel has no color, no smell, and really no taste for the most part. More importantly the product seems to work very well at helping to eliminate most gum problems. People report using the gel by putting a sizable dab on their toothbrush and then brushing their teeth with it. I suggest using the gel at night as a tooth gel and then use your choice of a good whitening toothpaste in the morning. Most people report that if they brush their teeth at night with the gel, when they wake up in the morning, their mouth is still squeaky clean, because no bad bacteria grew in their mouth overnight. If used in this way, most people report a very positive result against the gingivitis within just a few days to a week. By brushing your teeth with gel, the tooth brush helps push the gel product up into the gums were it can better help kill the pathogens and also help with the healing of the gums. As an extra bonus, the theory also makes sense that using the gel on your toothbrush will keep bacteria or other bad things from growing on the toothbrush, helping to eliminate another potential problem area.

A number of dentists also report using the 10 ppm Nano silver liquid as a mouthwash, especially after dental work has been completed, swishing it around in their mouths after they brush their teeth and then swallowing the liquid as an immune boosting supplement. When used as a mouthwash the liquid can help keep down the bacteria counts in the mouth and that will help keep new dental work from being infected (lowering the risk of secondary infections). If you do not like the taste of the gel many people will brush their teeth with the Nano silver liquid.

To really solve the problem I know that a new Nano silver based tooth gel has been engineered for the natural health market. The new tooth gel includes not only the Nano silver gel but also xylitol, and peppermint oil. Three natural bacteria killing ingredients together for the first time. I expect that new silver tooth gel will do amazing things for the health of teeth and gums!

## GONORRHEA

The data still surprises me, but in a report I read from human case studies in Africa, the doctors reported that they treated two cases of Gonorrhea. The report stated that the patients were taking two teaspoons, two times daily. It went on to state that the two patients showed signs of recovery in just 3.5 days and were what the doctors deemed as fully recovered in just six days.

## HAND SANITIZER

In a hand scrub study it was found that the 24 ppm Nano silver gel could give the skin a layer of protection that would last for about 4 hours. In other words, in the test it showed that rubbing the gel on the skin killed all the bad bacteria the skin came in contact with for a period of about four hours, like a hand sanitizer but better. A hand sanitizer just kills the bacteria that are on the skin at that moment. Most have almost no ability to kill bacteria or anything else on an ongoing basis, so with a regular hand sanitizer, as soon as you touch something new after using it, your hands are reinfected with the bacteria, etc. The 24 ppm Nano silver gel pulls into the outer layers of the skin, making it incredibly soft but also giving the skin a barrier of antibacterial protection that lasts for hours, until it wears off. You can tell when it wears off because the skin will no longer have that incredibly soft feeling. The 24 ppm gel does not cause skin irritation, is not toxic, and will not harm a person if accidently swallowed, unlike some other hand sanitizers that are poisonous if swallowed, especially by a child.

The potential hand sanitizer alternative use is very important, especially for people who work out in a gym and must touch machines and weights that other people have just used and sweated on. It can also be used on the hands when you have to touch a grocery shopping cart, public handrail, tray on a plane, daycare, school, or anything at all in a hospital setting, etc.

## HAIR GEL AND HEAD RUB

See dandruff treatment above.

## HEMORRHOIDS

Hemorrhoids are an inflammation of the veins. As they stick out, they can become sore and problematic. As a pleasant surprise, I started to receive reports from people, especially weight lifters, who reported a very positive effect the gel was having on hemorrhoids. They reported that just by putting the 24 ppm Nano silver gel on the affected area, the inflammation was going away and the hemorrhoids were gone in only a week or two. The protocol was to cover the hemorrhoids with the gel three times daily. In my own case, I tried it and mine were gone within the first week and have never returned. Hopefully you will have similar results.

## HEPATITIS B/C

Hepatitis is a deadly disease. It makes people very sick and kills many of them. Long term viral infections are much harder to treat than bacterial infections. A number of in vitro tests have shown that the Nano silver liquid can neutralize virus. I have known of four people who have sent me data on their blood test work who are infected with the Hepatitis c. virus. Almost all of them are reporting similar results against the virus.

They reported that they are drinking six teaspoons of the 10 ppm Nano silver liquid product every day, spread throughout the day. Almost all are reporting that over a period of about 30-45 days, they are able to cut down by half the viral load they have in their bodies. It doesn't really seem to matter what the viral numbers start at, about half of it is eliminated in that first 30-45 days. They have then been reporting that about another half of the remaining viral load is again eliminated in the next 30-45 days of daily use by taking the product at the same level. So about 75% of their viral load was eliminated within the first 60-90 days.

The problem then became that in all four cases the person started to feel so good that they stopped taking the product for a period of time, or only took it sporadically, and then the viral load slowly began to build back up. Time will tell if we can help the body to eliminate the virus completely, but I can say that it would seem that we can definitely help the people to feel better and live much more productive lives. We have a report of a cranky old military man who said that his doctors sent him home to die, saying that they had done all they could for him. He started using the product and reported that he can now golf again and feels great. He did not bother to get his blood checked, but uses the product every day and said that he now feels much better. Again, I do not know if the virus is still in his system, but at the least he is now able to function and enjoy life.

My belief is that in the years to come the protocols will be established and clinical tests will be finished that will show that use by injection or IV's, of the 10 ppm Nano silver will help to eliminate deadly virus from the blood possibly as fast as within the first month of treatment. My belief is that the 10 ppm Nano silver product will probably work at a use level of approximately 10 mil/BD/ every third or fourth day, for a 30 day period. Actual viral load numbers, when checked, will quickly establish if the protocol is working or not, and adjustments could then be made. I believe that by perfecting this type of use protocol, millions of lives will be saved, and potentially huge hospital and medical costs will be reduced or eliminated. I believe that it will be found that the buffer will need to be a D5W or other non-saline buffer additive. I believe that this type of protocol, once perfected, may work to help eliminate numerous deadly viral diseases. I also believe that the Nano silver liquid could also be jointly used with other antivirals (if needed) like AZT, Ribavirin or Interferon to have a dual action attack on the viral diseases. The drugs could be used at lower levels which will also help reduce the nasty side effects associated with the use of these types of drugs.

# HIV (AIDS)

I do not know that all forms of silver will neutralize virus, but the 10 ppm Nano silver has without a doubt been proven to neutralize many different viruses including HIV, but it does take a little time to function. In a preliminary test against a bacteria eating virus, the 10 ppm Nano silver liquid was able to neutralize a billion virus in about 2.5 hours of contact time. The key is that the silver Nano particles has to have access to the virus - it does not just magically disappear or die off. In the case of HIV, the virus infects the white blood cells (T lymphocyte). I am not sure if the silver actually makes it directly into the T cells—that still needs to be tested—or if it just neutralizes the virus once a virus filled cell ruptures and the new virus is released into the bloodstream to search for more white cells.

A peer review published human ingestion study was released to the public [9] in 2008 showing the dramatic impact the 10 ppm Nano silver can have on AIDS patients. The study, labeled as a preliminary study, was the editor's note on an in vivo H5N1 study that was published using the Nano silver as well. The editors of the journal decided that if the 10 ppm Nano silver worked against the H5N1 bird flu just by drinking it, it should work against the AIDS virus. The study was completed by a number of top U.S. and Indian scientists who worked together on the project, and once published, the results were also picked up and published by CNBC News. In the 7-person human trial, the AIDS patients drank 2 ounces daily of a 10 ppm Nano silver product, split into three doses (TID). It was reported that within two weeks of starting on the silver, all the patients regained their appetites, and over a 4 month period of time they were able to gain an average of about 17.6 pounds of body weight; a miracle in and of itself. There are currently a number of FDA cleared drugs that just help AIDS patients gain weight. More importantly, the AIDS patients were able to achieve an average T cell increase of about 39.54% over the 4 month period of the study time. In other words, the silver Nano particles helped all the patients to rebuild their immune systems and regain their health.

The viral load counts of the patients were not released as part of the study, but I was personally told by the authors that the viral counts in the blood dropped like a rock, meaning that they had a very significant reduction in the amount of virus left in the bloodstream. As a side note, I have an email from a man telling me that after using a 10 ppm Nano silver for an extended period of time, he now tests negative for the disease. I believe that is entirely possible to achieve with the Nano silver treatment.

I believe that given the current information we have available to us, a cure for AIDS certainly could be developed using the silver Nano particles. Oral use, I believe will do it, but it will take an extended period of use to help that happen. However, I also believe that injection and IV protocols could easily be developed that could eliminate the virus from the body within as little as 30 days. Because direct application of the silver right into the blood stream would put the silver Nano particles in direct contact with the virus at a faster rate, neutralizing the virus and helping the immune system to overcome the disease. I think a non-saline buffer would have to be used to cut the silver, my guess is that a 50/50 ratio with a D5W would do.

Unfortunately, I think the only thing keeping those protocols from being developed right now is the political climate and also the huge money being poured into big pharma companies for HIV drugs that do not cure but only treat symptoms. To cure the disease would mean an end to the money stream accrued by these companies on an annual basis. I hope I am wrong and they will soon be established, but based on the political treatment of the information produced so far, and the big money associated with only treating the symptoms, I cannot see that the powers that be can let an HIV cure happen.

## HPV (VAGINAL PAPILLOMA VIRUS INFECTION)

HPV is an STD that can and does affect many women worldwide. Numerous case studies have been reported saying that the 24 ppm gel can have a miraculous impact on this disease. HPV can reside in sores or lesions that develop on the face of the cervix. It is believed that HPV can lead to cervical cancer if left untreated. Reports indicate that the possible protocol for treatment includes a two-step process. First douche with the 10 ppm Nano silver liquid. Then by use of a vaginal applicator, introduce two teaspoons or 10 mil. of the 24 ppm Nano silver gel into the vaginal canal at the face of the cervix. Repeat twice daily. Use at bedtime is very important as it gives the silver all night to work with little interruption. Positive results have also been reported placing the 5-10 ml. of gel on a tampon and inserting it into the vagina and leaving it in for the entire night. Very positive results have been reported in as little as two weeks, with no reported negative side effects.

## INFLAMMATION OF THE JOINTS:

Laboratory personnel have noted that in addition to its ability to kill bacteria and inhibit the growth of yeasts, the 10 ppm Nano Silver liquid is a powerful anti-inflammatory agent. Researchers have suggested that this may be one of the reasons that the pain from conditions like earaches and canker sores recedes so quickly. In order to informally test this theory, one researcher donated a bottle of 10 ppm Nano liquid to a young woman suffering from fibromyalgia, which causes a painful swelling in the joints and also the muscle tissue. She reported that after using one teaspoon per day, for one week, she was able to reduce her joint pain medication by 90%. She claimed that almost all the swelling was gone from the joints and also that her energy level had dramatically improved. I would think that if I were the one establishing the protocol I would have had her use two teaspoons, three times daily, but it would be hard to argue the point, since she claimed that what she did worked well for her. I also had a grandma that used the 10 ppm Nano liquid to help reduce the inflammation in her joints. She died a natural death at age 94. But before she died she used the 10 ppm daily to reduce the inflammation in her joints. She said that use of the product did not repair the damaged cartilage but that it seemed to help her to move a lot easier in the morning without having to "warm up her joints". I believe it was the anti-inflammatory effect of the silver Nano particles that helped her. When I asked her how much was drinking daily she said she took a "glug" out of the bottle. I am not sure I know exactly how much a "glug" is, but from what she described I believe it to be around 1-2 ounces daily.

## INJECTION AND IV THERAPY

I believe that Nano silver has the ability to eliminate both virus and bacterial infections from the bloodstream. A published human study has already shown that the 10 ppm Nano silver has no negative impact on the blood platelets.[20] I believe that sepsis (blood poisoning) can be eliminated from the blood in as little as a single day by injection therapy. As stated above (see Hep. C.) My belief is that in the years to come, the protocols will be established and clinical tests will be finished, that will show that use by injection or IV's, of the 10 ppm Nano silver liquid, the silver will help to eliminate deadly virus from the blood stream in as little as the first 30 days of treatment.

Actual viral load numbers, when routinely checked, will quickly establish if the protocol is working or not, adjustments could then be made. I believe that by perfecting this type of use protocol, millions of lives will be saved, and potentially huge hospital and medical costs will be reduced or eliminated. I believe that it will be found that the buffer will need to be a D5W or other non-saline buffer additive at a 50/50 dilution. I believe that the silver liquid could also be jointly used with other antivirals (if needed) like AZT, Ribavirin, or Interferon, to have a dual action attack on the deadly viral diseases. The drugs could be used at lower levels which will also help reduce the nasty side effects associated with the use of these types of drugs.

In a book on silver one doctor stated, "There is a very experimental method for IV usage. About 3,000 cases have used Silver Sol intravenously, with no reported toxicity problems. An IV can be made utilizing 250 CCs of Silver Sol liquid at 10 parts per million. Mix one to one with a D5W mixture hung in a bag and dripped for one hour, given every other day for 10 total doses."[23]

## ITCH

I have probably used the product to alleviate an itch on my skin a thousand times. From allergic reactions to plants, to bug bites, to the itch of a past sunburn starting to peel. I have used it on my arms, hands, legs, and even my face. It never fails to alleviate the itch within minutes. I have had dozens of other people report the same findings. All you have to do is to apply the 24 ppm Nano silver gel to the area of the skin that itches. As I said above, the itch will usually go away within just a few minutes.

## JELLY FISH STING

Jelly fish stings can be very painful but are rarely ever fatal. The 24 ppm Nano silver gel seems to help take the pain out of the sting, usually within 15-30 minutes of contact time. Liberally cover the affected area of the skin with a layer of the 24 ppm Nano sliver gel. Reapply as needed. It is believed that the silver Nano particle steals the electrons off the toxic protein chains, precipitating out or eliminating the toxic nature of the chains and making them benign or non-irritating or problematic. Simply apply the 24 ppm gel to the affected area as needed.

## JOCK ITCH

Jock itch seems to be easily taken care of with the help of the 24 ppm Nano silver gel. Simply liberally apply the Nano silver gel to the affected area as needed to help soothe the burn and itch and help heal the rash. It is especially effective to apply the 24 ppm Nano silver gel just before bedtime, because it gives the gel all night to work.

## LARYNGITIS

Spray on rear of throat and gargle with at least 1 tablespoon of the 10 ppm Nano silver liquid, three to four times per day. Expect relief in one to three days. If the laryngitis is accompanied by a sore throat, see the section on "sore throat" below.

## LIVER PROBLEMS

For some reason that has never been adequately explained, Nano silver seems to have a very positive effect on the health and function of the liver. There is no question that Nano silver helps the liver immensely to perform its functions, the question is how it does it? In one case study a friend of mine in Las Vegas had another friend with a serious drinking problem. This drinking problem had caused a significant negative impact on his liver (cirrhosis). The man had tested his liver and found that it was on the verge of a shutdown. After two months of using about an ounce daily (two teaspoons three times daily) he again had the doctor test his liver. The doctor told him that his liver was again functioning at a very high level, and he was very much surprised and ask him what he was taking, he told him.

In another report a person sent me information on their dog. The dog had had a serious liver disease and his liver function had dropped to about 25%. The dog owners were dismayed when the vet told them that the dog would not probably last long and would probably die of a blood infection. At that point the dog owners put the dog on the silver at a level of about an ounce a day, just putting it in his water dish. They said the dog seemed to like the taste of it and would just lap it up from his bowl. They reported that the dog had had his good days and his bad days but was still alive and kicking three years after the vet had told them he did not have long to live.

## LYME DISEASE

Lyme disease is a horrible and debilitating disease. Antibiotics are usually used to treat it and the treatment can last years, because the Lyme disease spirochete can hide in the tissue if it is under attack, and then build up again once the person stops taking antibiotics. It is very difficult to get rid of. There was a nurse that came to us and told us that her daughter had been suffering from Lyme disease for nine years. The nurse said that she had tried to treat the child for years with antibiotics and the girl still had the disease. The woman stated that it got so bad that they could not even touch the girl without causing her pain. She asked if we had any data on the treatment of Lyme disease and we told her that we did not. We told her that we would supply her with the product if she wanted to try it. She said that she did and would keep a record and make a report for us whether the information was good or bad on the effectiveness of the product. She started giving her daughter six teaspoons of a 10 ppm Nano silver product every day. She stated that for the first week or so her daughter became even sicker. (This is not uncommon and is called a Herxsheimer effect.) After the first week of taking the silver product, her daughter started to get better.

Do not overdose the person with the silver, because a big over dose of the silver can kill too many of the spirochetes, releasing too much toxin at once, which can cause the person to become extremely ill. After about 30 days the girl was doing much better and began to recover to the point where she could function normally. After a few months the girl was able to go back to school and get a new job. Over a period of a year the girl seemed to recover fully. The girl has now been married with children and seems to be doing very well.

Over the years I have seen many other cases of people who have taken the product to fend off the disease and it seems to work for them as well. One man who goes to the doctor to have his blood checked, told me that after using the product for several years the doctor reported that the disease has now been eliminated from his blood stream. I do not know if it is really gone or not, but I guess that what matters is that he can live his life and function without the pain or sickness of the disease. I have been getting many such personal reports.

Some doctors are using the silver in combination with herbs and other natural antimicrobial products. Very good reports also come from these doctors and the combined therapy also seems to be great especially for patients with advanced symptoms. Again however, you may want to start slowly so that the patient's liver has time to filter out the toxins and dead pathogens, and this will minimize the increased sickness or Herxsheimer effect.

## MALARIA

Malaria is the second leading cause of death by infection on the earth today. The sickness is caused by one of four different parasites that are injected into the blood by the bite of a mosquito. Malaria currently kills 3,000 children a day in Africa (Nairobi AP article, 4/28/03). The ten ppm Nano silver liquid has been shown to be incredibly effective in eliminating the parasite from the blood stream. The protocol for use is to take two teaspoons of the 10 ppm Nano silver liquid three times daily (morning, noon, and night).

Reports from a published peer review journal article[7] outline the use of a 10 ppm Nano silver product in 56 human case studies from four different African hospitals and clinics. The report showed that the product eliminated the parasite from the blood in an average of 3.43 days, with patients walking out of the hospital fully recovered in 4-5 days on average.

The report goes on to state that there were no treatment failures and that all patients fully recovered. Patients in the case studies ranged in age from 1year old, to over 90 years old. The report lists the product as a cure not just a treatment. In 2005, Congress requested a copy of the data in the form of a full US Congressional Committee Testimony, under the direction of Chairman Smith. At the same time the data was given to the WHO and the Roll Back Malaria committee or foundation, who subsequently did nothing with the data.

It has become my belief that these groups do not want an answer to be found for the disease, because that would eliminate the billions of dollars they receive from governments and private people to work on it. I believe that Malaria is also being used as a way to help control the population growth in many of these countries.

## MASSAGE THERAPY

The 24 ppm Nano silver gel is a great product for massage therapy for a number of reasons. First, if the patient smells bad (has body odor) the gel can be rubbed onto the patient so that the gel can kill the odor causing bacteria. The Nano silver gel will kill the odor causing bacteria within about 10 minutes. Secondly, because it is a hydrogel, the 24 ppm Nano silver gel will make the skin feel amazingly soft in about 2 minutes, which is desirable for both the patient's skin and also the hands of the massage therapist. Third, hand scrub studies show that the silver gel will kill bacteria on the skin for about 4 hours, allowing the therapist to have a layer of protection between him or her and the patient which they have to touch.

## MASTITIS

Mastitis is a painful inflammation in the breast. Nursing mothers may be hesitant to take antibiotics while nursing their babies. It has been reported that using two teaspoons three times a day of the 10 ppm silver Nano particle liquid, has helped clear up mastitis in as little as two days.

The 24 ppm gel can also help heal cracked or sore nipples, while having no toxic effect on the feeding baby.

## MOLDS AND ENVIRONMENTAL FUNGI

There are numerous forms of mold and fungus that can not only infect your house, but can also get into your lungs and cause some severe respiratory tract infections. The Nano silver liquid at 10 ppm has been shown to effectively kill numerous types of mold and fungus.[26] The 10 ppm Nano silver liquid can be used in a nebulizer for 5–10 minutes, three or four times daily. If you detect the mold or fungus growing in your house or office, spray the silver solution directly on the affected area, thoroughly soaking it and leaving it in contact for at least 15 minutes before wiping it off.

## MOUTH WASH

Use the 10 ppm Nano silver liquid as a mouthwash. A number of dentists have determined that the antibacterial nature of the silver 10 ppm liquid makes it a perfect disinfectant for a mouth wash and also after dental work. To use simply put about three teaspoons of silver in your mouth and swish around for several minutes, working it between teeth if you can. You can then swallow it if you would like to, to help boost the immune system. It will usually help reduce the redness and inflammation of the gums and also help promote healthy gums and teeth.

## PERIODONTAL DISEASE

The Nano silver gel has been used with positive effect for periodontal disease. Brush your teeth with the 24 ppm Nano silver gel at least once a day. Positive change has been noticed within one to two weeks. Another form of effective treatment is to put the 10 ppm Nano silver liquid into a water pick sprayer or water flosser and spray directly into the gum lines. The sprayer will force the liquid silver up under the gums where it can directly kill the bacteria and help shrink the perio-pockets. Dentists are reporting very quick recovery times and also reattachment of the gums to the teeth (shrinking the pockets). This treatment is especially effective if you go to the dentist first for a cleaning and scaling of the affected areas and then start treatment with the silver afterwards.

# PERSONAL LUBRICANT

A published article listed the 24 ppm Nano silver gel as a very good personal lubricant. There are many reasons why the 24 ppm gel makes a good personal lubricant. First, it has a very slick feel that lasts only a few minutes, making entry easier on the female, but not leaving a greasy or slimy feel. Second, because it is antimicrobial the gel can kill yeast and bacteria in the vagina, helping to protect both partners. In test tube tests, the gel also neutralized virus, which it has also been theorized to do in the vaginal tract, meaning that there is a real potential that the gel could help protect sexual partners against a number of STD's (sexually transmitted diseases).

A series of tests showed that although the gel was effective at killing bacteria and yeast, it did no harm to the vaginal probiotics. In other words, the gel killed the bad bacteria but not the good or helpful bacteria. The article also said that the gel, if vaginally applied could eliminate a vaginal yeast infection within 90 minutes.

# PNEUMONIA

Pneumonia is caused by the growth of either bacteria or virus in the lungs. The good news is that Nano silver can kill or neutralize both. The most effective way to use the silver to help combat pneumonia is to use a nebulizer. A nebulizer is a small machine that takes a liquid and makes it into a cold mist so that it can be easily breathed in. They are used a lot to get medicine into the lungs of kids with asthma, but they are also great to use with the Nano silver liquid. To use, simply put one to two teaspoons of the Nano silver liquid into the little liquid holding bowel, turn the machine on and breathe in the cool mist. You could do it while watching TV, etc. For use to help fight against pneumonia, repeat three to four times daily. The nebulizer will help get full strength product directly on the problem bug or pathogen in the lungs. I have heard of cases where people have reported that they were able to overcome pneumonia in as little as two days using the Nano silver liquid in a nebulizer. I would also suggest drinking two teaspoons of the 10 ppm Nano silver liquid three times daily, to help boost the body's entire immune system, while it fights the lung infection.

Pneumonia is also the number one killer of people in comas in hospitals. The pathogens can get in through the breathing machines and grow quickly, killing the patients. I have studied the problem and believe there may be an easy answer to it. The hospital breathing machines have a humidifier attached which adds a cool mist into the breathing machine. I think that it is possible to just replace the regular water with the 10 ppm Nano silver in the humidifier and let the silver do its job to kill the bacteria before it can grow in the breathing tubes and lungs. I think that even if it were only done every few days it could make a huge difference in saving the lives of thousands of hospital coma patients and it would have no negative effect.

## POISON OAK/IVY TREATMENT

When you touch poison oak or ivy the resin from the plant gets on your skin and probably your clothes. The resin does not easily come off the clothes and can re-infect more skin it comes in contact with, and possibly spread to other clothes if you try to wash the toxins out. Do not wash affected clothes, just throw them away - it is not worth the possible continued problems. Skin contact with the resin and can cause pain, blistering and sores that can last for weeks. You need to put the gel on as soon as possible. The longer the resin is on the skin, the more damage it can do.

The good news is that the 24 ppm Nano silver gel seems to help eliminate many of the symptoms (the itch and burn) usually within 30 minutes of contact time. Liberally cover the affected area of the skin with a layer of the 24 ppm Nano sliver gel. Reapply as needed, but at least three times daily, until the problem is resolved. It is believed that the silver Nano particle steals the electrons off the toxic protein chains, precipitating out or eliminating the toxic nature of the protein chains and making them benign, non-irritating, or problematic.

## POST DERMABRASION AND MICRODERMABRASION

Dermabrasion and microdermabrasion are techniques that damage the skin in a controlled way, scraping or cutting off layers of the skin to cause the body to produce new tissue or skin. It is done many times to reduce scaring from acne, remove wrinkles, remove tattoos etc.. The result is damage to the skin area that can be painful, red and inflamed. After the treatment has been completed, the 24 ppm can be used to reduce the redness, inflammation and pain. It will also help heal the damaged skin usually in about half the normal time. To use, simply cover the affected area liberally with the 24 ppm nano silver gel at least 2–3 times a day or as often is needed.

## POST PEELING

Post peeling is very similar to dermabrasion, in the fact that damage is done to the skin to promote new healthy skin growth. Two of the methods for peeling the skin would be to use chemical peels or a laser, both of which are used to remove layers of the skin by burning it off. The theory is that then the new skin would be cleaner, brighter and healthier. Either way the skin ends up burned, red and sore. The 24 ppm Nano silver gel is the perfect answer to help with many of the problems associated with the repair of the skin and the cooling relief of the pain from the burn. As stated above, simply cover the affected area liberally with the 24 ppm nano silver gel at least 2–3 times a day or as often is needed. Recovery will usually happen in about half the normal time using the silver gel.

## POST WAXING OR HAIR REMOVAL

Hair removal from the legs, body or face can be painful. Using products like hot wax, tape, honey, or glue products can leave the skin red, raw, and painful. Hot wax can also burn the skin. Treating the problem is really easy. Just liberally apply the 24 ppm Nano silver gel to the affected area. Usually the pain and redness will subside in just minutes. Recently, I attended an international aesthetician conference and found that one of the top suppliers of hair removal wax products actually sold a 24 ppm Nano silver product right out of the booth with the wax products, the owner of the business said the Nano silver was the best product on the market to use after waxing.

## RADIATION BURNS

A thousand-bottle radiation burn study was completed using the product at a large cancer clinic. Because radiation is an important part of cancer treatment and because the use of radiation causes burns, a study was completed using first the 10 ppm liquid Nano silver and then later the 24 ppm Nano silver gel. The gel product was found to be superior to the use of just the liquid in treating the burns. The 24 ppm Nano silver gel was applied to the burned area 3–6 times daily.

In the report, the gel was found to first, deliver an instantaneous cooling effect that greatly helped sooth the burn. Secondly, the Nano silver gel was found to promote much faster healing and recovery than was anticipated—about half the normal time. Also, when used prophylactically (meaning that the gel was put on the skin before the cancer treatment had happened) the product was found to delay the onset of radiation-induced epidermitis and mucusitis.

In addition, the doctor reported that the product was found effective at treating other types of burns, including chemotherapy, and fire or heat induced burns. No adverse or negative effects were found in the use of the product on the burns. In fact, the doctor noted that, "two thirds of the patients rave about the product and ask for more as long as the problem for which it is given exists!" Because the 24 ppm Nano silver gel has been shown to be non-toxic in numerous safety tests, it has a strategic advantage over other burn care products, because it can be used orally to treat burns inside the mouth and throat where other products cannot be used. This information may become much more important as the world continues to have more and more natural disasters and man caused problems. Because the gel lasts for at least three years, it can also be put in emergency storage supplies.

## RASHES

Rashes are usually easily taken care of with the use of the 24 ppm Nano silver gel. Apply the gel liberally to the affected area. Usually the burning and itch from the rash will be eliminated within minutes (15–30) and the rash is usually healed up within a few days.

# RETRO VIRAL INFECTION

In the first human study, an HIV patient was sick with a retro viral infection. The suggested use is two teaspoons, three times daily. In the study the doctors reported that the patient showed signs of recovery in 4 days and was deemed as fully recovered from the infection (not the AIDS) in just five days.

# SCARS

The 24 ppm Nano silver gel is very helpful in healing scar tissue, but it takes time for it to work on old scars. The gel will not kill or have any negative effect on human tissue so it only replaces the old scar tissue when that skin cell naturally dies. So as you use the gel daily on the old scars and those skin cells die, new non-scar tissue replaces it, thus minimizing the scar. Over time many scars become so faint they are almost not seen unless a person looks very closely. One doctor I know had a rather big scar on his face, and application of the gel to the scar area daily, over a period of a year, minimized it to the point you really could not see it any more.

The best way to prevent a scar from forming is to use the gel on the wound when it happens and also continuing to use it afterword. That way when the wound heals it is already forming the new tissue and the scaring is very much minimized. One man I know had an open heart surgery and the gel was used in the closing of the wound and also afterwards. When the wound was healed you could hardly even see where his chest had been split open - it was amazingly clean new pink tissue.

# SHAVING (ESPECIALLY SENSITIVE AREAS)/RAZOR BURN

Using the 24 ppm gel, cover the area to be shaved with a thin layer of the gel. The gel will provide a wonderful lubricating cover to the skin which will aid in the closeness of the save. The gel will help protect sensitive shaving areas, reducing razor burn and making the skin feel soft and wonderful. The gel easily washes out of the hand held razors with just the warm water from the tap.

# SHINGLES

Shingles are caused by the same virus that causes chicken pox, they just usually happen in older people as they get stressed and their immune system weakens. Shingles are easily identified by red itching or burning spots or rash looking areas. The 24 ppm Nano silver gel seems to help greatly to reduce the itching and burning associated with the rash or spots. Simply liberally apply the silver gel to the affected areas and usually relief will be evident within 20-30 minutes, reducing both the pain and itch. It is also theorized that internal use of the liquid will also help reduce the duration of the shingles break out. I believe that use of both the liquid and the gel may also help reduce or knock down the amount of the virus that is in the body.

# SINUS INFECTIONS

There were six sinus infections reported in one group of human case studies, released in information presented to Congress at their request. The information was subsequently released by the Congressional Record. (17) In the report, the doctors said that they were putting the 10 ppm product into the nasal passages three time daily. They reported that they were treating both Sinusitis and Rhinitis. The doctors reported that the patients showed signs of recovery on the second day and were deemed as fully recovered on average by the third day. One of the patients had stated that he had had sinus infections for 10 years and it was now gone in just three days. I had a medical doctor call me from Arizona to tell me that the product had worked a miracle in his sinuses in just a few days and that he was now recommending it to all his patients. To use, irrigate with one-half teaspoon per nostril, three times per day. Relief can be noticeable in 24 hours, with complete remission often occurring within two to three days.

# SORE THROAT

Both the antibacterial and the anti-inflammatory properties of silver solution may help play a role in its effect on sore throats. To use, take one to two tablespoons into mouth, and gargle for 4-5 minutes-swallow. Repeat at least 2-3 times daily. We have had reports of people saying that they were using the product and that the sore throat was going away, but that it was coming back over night. We found that the problem was that the infecting agent may have actually been located in the sinus area and that even if it was killed in the throat, it was still being re-infected by liquid dripping from the sinus cavity at night. We found that the answer to the problem was to also spray or drip some solution into the nasal passages and that seemed to end the problem.

Another remarkable find was that by swallowing a mouth full of the 24 ppm Nano silver gel just before going to bed, after everything else has been done (like brushing teeth or drinking water etc.), the gel coats the throat. By coating the throat, the gel has a much longer time to work before it is washed away by eating or drinking. The gel also seems to have a very soothing effect on the pain making it much easier for a sick child to sleep. By treating a sore throat with both the liquid and the gel, most people are reporting very noticeable improvements within 12–48 hours.

## STINKY FEET

The stink part of stinky feet, is usually caused by odor causing bacteria growing on the feet. By simply spraying the 10 ppm Nano silver liquid on the feet or rubbing the feet down with the 24 ppm Nano silver gel, the silver can usually kill the odor causing bacteria within minutes. Killing the bacteria will usually eliminate the stinky smell within 10–30 minutes.

For really stubborn cases of stink, you may want to dilute down the 10 ppm Nano silver liquid half and half with store purchased hydrogen peroxide (it is usually sold at a 3% strength), the mix of the silver and the hydrogen peroxide (5 ppm silver, 1.5 % hydrogen peroxide) when sprayed on the feet, makes a dual-action product that can really be effective for eliminating the stink quickly.

## SUNBURN

Sunburns are a very painful type of skin burn. The 24 ppm Nano silver gel seems to do an incredible job when it comes to sun burns and also the pain associated with the sunburn. It is really important to use the silver as soon as possible (ASAP) after the burn happens. The silver gel should be used as many as three times in the first three hours (once every hour) to help stop the burn from continuing to destroy tissue, to help eliminate the heat from the burn, and to start the healing process. Leave the product on and let it dry. The anti-inflammatory nature of the silver metal seems to be the factor in helping to reduce the pain.

In tests at a major cancer clinic that used the Nano silver gel for the burns associated with radiation treatment, the doctor stated that the patients reported that the silver gel caused an instantaneous cooling effect on the burns. He also stated that the burns were healing in about half the normal time, with much reduced pain (a sunburn is actually just a type of radiation burn). To continue to treat a burn after the initial treatment has been completed, continue to liberally use the silver gel on the sunburned area of skin as needed, at least 2-3 times a day, until the burn has recovered.

I have personally used a 24 ppm Nano silver gel for sun burns and found it to be very effective in helping to treat the burns and in helping to reduce the pain. My skin still peeled about four days after I received the burn, and as the skin pealed the area started to itch and it was driving me crazy. I again reapplied the Nano silver gel on the part of my skin that itched and within minutes the itch was gone.

## TATTOO OR POST TATTOO REMOVAL

The art of tattooing is to use needles to put ink under layers of the skin so that it stays there on a permanent basis spelling words or forming pictures. Some are amazing pieces of art that are very intricately designed. Because it is created using a needle that penetrates the skin hundreds or even thousands of times, there is a very good potential to get bacterial infections of the skin which can not only ruin the art, it can make the person very sick. In one surgical hand scrub study, a 24 ppm Nano silver gel was found to disinfect the skin for about four hours. With that in mind the 24 ppm Nano silver gel can be used on the skin before tattooing to clean the area and to kill bacteria. After the tattoo is finished the gel can be reapplied to help heal the puncture wounds caused by the tattoo needles.

Another big area is tattoo removal. Some people find that they no longer want the name of their ex-girlfriend or boyfriend etc. etc. tattooed on some part of their body and they wish to get it removed. One of the removal procedures is to use a laser to burn the skin, which brings the ink up to the surface of the skin. After the burn is completed and the ink has been brought up to the surface in the removal process, the gel can be used to heal the wound, but you have to wait about 24 hours before using the Nano silver gel to heal the post tattoo burn. If the gel is used too quickly after the treatment, it can heal the skin too quickly and the ink does not come to the surface as it is supposed to. So if you use the gel too quickly after the tattoo removal procedure, the procedure will not work.

## TOOTH DECAY

The silver product at just 10 ppm has been proven very effective at killing a number of the bacteria that are believed to cause tooth decay. Those same bacteria can also travel from the mouth down to the heart and cause valve problems, like endocarditis. So, if you take good care of your teeth with the Nano silver you may also be helping to keep your heart healthy. Not to mention the fact that if you use the 10 ppm Nano Silver liquid as a mouth wash after you brush your teeth, I believe that it may further help reduce tooth decay and also kill the bacteria that causes bad breath. For use in mouth, take one to two teaspoons into mouth, swish the solution around in your mouth for 4-5 minutes then swallow.

A lot of people are also using the 24 ppm Nano silver gel as a tooth-paste, it has almost no taste but it seems to do some really great things for the gums and teeth. One man told me that he knows that it works because when he wakes up in the morning after having used the silver at night, he doesn't have that film of gunk on his teeth that he normally has when he wakes up. To use the gel as a tooth gel simply put the 24 ppm gel on your toothbrush and brush away like you normally would, spit and rinse. I have been told that it can help wipe out gingivitis in just days. I have also heard a rumor that a new Nano silver tooth gel has hit the market, adding the triple power of Nano silver with both xylitol and peppermint oil, which are also both natural antimicrobials.

The brilliance of that product is that all three ingredients are natural bacteria killing machines. I am guessing that the good side effect from the use of the silver on the toothbrush is that it would also help keep bacteria from growing on the toothbrush. Another good side effect, is that I believe that because some of the toothpaste will be swallowed as you brush, I believe that it will also help kill H. pylori bacteria in the stomach, which is the bacteria responsible for causing stomach ulcers. So in essence I believe that the tooth gel will eliminate stomach ulcers.

## TOENAIL FUNGUS

A well-regarded, veteran, east-coast podiatrist treated one patient with mycotic toenails with the 10 ppm Nano Silver liquid. The results were so sufficiently impressive over a four-month period that he has begun treating others with this solution. File the shine off the toenail (to increase porosity) and then spray the solution directly on the infected toenail. For best results apply (saturate) a cotton ball with the 10 ppm liquid, tape onto the toenail and leave for up to 30 minutes. Repeat two or three times daily. Good results have been noted in as little as 30-40 days which is about half the time required by some of the antibiotics often prescribed for this condition.

If the person has less treatment time available to them, the 24 ppm gel can be used. After filing the shine off the toenail as described above, liberally cover the top of the toenail with the gel, wait a few minutes before putting on a sock.

## TONSILLITIS

Tonsillitis is harder to treat than some of the other conditions. It is harder because it is harder to keep the silver on the area long enough to kill the pathogens. In one case that was reported, the doctors said that they had the patient gargle with two teaspoons of the 10 ppm Nano silver liquid three times daily. They reported that the patient showed signs of recovery in just two days, but that it had taken seven days to achieve full recovery. I would add that it would have probably helped if they had also had the patient use some of the 10 ppm Nano silver liquid in his or her sinuses at the same time, because of the potential to help eliminate reinfection from the back of the sinuses. I think it also helps greatly to have the patient make sure to gargle right before bed after having completed all their other before bed nighttime tasks, like brushing the teeth, so that as the person goes to sleep, the silver might have a slightly longer contact time on the tonsils before it gets washed off. To use, gargle with two teaspoons three times daily. Gargle as long as possible (3–4 minutes if possible) and then swallow.

Most people report signs of recovery in about two days and full recovery in about a week. For people who can eat the almost no flavor 24 ppm Nano silver gel, it may really help to swallow a couple teaspoons of the gel right before bed time. By doing this, the gel can help coat the throat and have a lot more time to work overnight, which may lead to a faster recovery.

## TOYS (DISINFECTION)

Because the 10 ppm Nano silver is not toxic, has no smell, colors, or other nasty chemicals, it could be used to disinfect toys used by children, especially in a daycare center where toys are used by numerous different children every day. Many children's toys are covered with bacteria and are put directly into the mouths of the kids and so need to be disinfected. Soap residue can cause diarrhea and chemical disinfectants can be toxic and poisonous to children. The 10 ppm Nano silver is not toxic if ingested, so toys could be sprayed and left to dry, killing the bacteria and causing no damage to either the children or the non-porous hard plastic toys. Porous material like soft cotton, could be discolored if the silver is sprayed on and then left to dry. Hard plastics are not affected.

## THRUSH

It is common for little children to become infected with thrush in their mouths, especially if they are breast feeding. I suggest that you place several drops of the 10 ppm Nano silver liquid in each side of the child's mouth four times a day. There are reports of this condition in a young child clearing up in just two days. I also suggest that the mother use the 24 ppm Nano silver gel to help eliminate the thrush from her nipples, by liberally applying the gel to the nipples three times daily. Using the gel on the nipples may also help heal the nipples, if they become cracked or sore from breast feeding.

## TUBERCULOSIS (TB)

Tuberculosis is listed as the number one cause of death by infection on the earth today. It is a lung infection. TB spreads rapidly and kills millions of people annually. In the first set of direct in-vitro (test tube) tests, the 10 ppm silver Nano product was able to achieve a kill rate of 97.3 % in just 45 minutes of contact time. While this kill time is not overly fast, it is very significant! Because the silver is non-toxic when used in small amounts, a number of scientists that I work with have theorized that the product could be placed into a nebulizer and inhaled directly into the lungs.

Having already proven that the product could kill the TB bacteria, this theory would place the full strength 10 ppm Nano silver product directly on the TB bacteria in the lungs. With repeated use, huge amounts of the bacteria infecting the lungs could be directly contacted, and subsequently killed over a period of just a few days, without any negative side effects to the person using the silver. More work needs to be completed to prove that the theory will work on a large scale, but numerous individual doctor case studies report that it does work. I believe that with a 10 ppm Nano silver product and a nebulizer, millions of lives could easily be saved annually. The harder question is whether or not governments would let it happen and my guess is that many governments actually may, because TB is a poor man's disease and there is not a lot of money to be made by treating it. The current theory, based on limited case studies is that by using two teaspoons three times daily in the nebulizer, full recovery may be possible in as little as three days.

## ULCERS

Silver works incredibly well in helping to heal ulcers of many kinds. The 24 ppm Nano silver gel is amazing when used on skin ulcers. When you first start to treat the wound, it is probably best to wash out the wound first with the 10 ppm Nano silver liquid, which will help remove any debris and start killing any infective bacteria. The 24 ppm Nano silver gel can usually help heal many types of skin ulcers within just days, some take longer because of restricted blood flow, like diabetic ulcers. To use for general purposes, simply apply the gel liberally to the affected area and cover with a bandage or clean gauze wrap. Change out the bandage and reapply the gel at least once daily. Usually you will see good improvement within just a few days and healing of the wound will take about half the normal time.

Stomach ulcers are usually caused by a bacterial infection called H. pylori. The good news is that the silver Nano particle can easily kill the bug, the bad news is that it takes a few minutes for the silver to kill it and when the Nano silver liquid hits the stomach, it is pulled into the body through the stomach wall so fast it is not there long enough to kill it. There are probably two good ways to get the job done. One is to drink a little silver every few hours during the day several days in a row. The constant attack of the silver on the bacteria in the stomach is probably enough to get rid of the bacteria so the ulcer can heal. The other way to do it is to eat a teaspoon or two of the 24 ppm Nano silver gel three times daily for a few days. The gel takes longer to clear the stomach so it will be in contact with the bacteria for a longer period of time, thus making it easier to kill the bacteria, so that stomach lining can heal itself.

## UPPER RESPIRATORY TRACT INFECTIONS

There are numerous reports from people using the 10 ppm Nano silver for the treatment of upper respiratory tract infections. The suggested amount to use is to drink two teaspoons three times daily (morning, noon, night). Many doctors report that their patients are showing signs of recovery in three days and are gaining full recovery in about six days. To speed up the process, a number of doctors have started using the product in a nebulizer. A nebulizer is a small compressor that makes a liquid into a cold light mist. A lot of people with asthma own nebulizers and use them to receive medicine directly in the lungs. Nebulizers can be purchased from numerous sites online. The mist comes out of a tube and the tube is placed into the mouth so that the mist is breathed directly into the lungs. The nebulizer makes it so that a person can breathe in the Nano-silver particles directly into the lungs. By breathing in the silver liquid, the full strength silver Nano particles can have direct access to the pathogen (bacteria, mold, or virus) causing problems in the lungs, and can kill or neutralize them faster. Some doctors are reporting that using the nebulizer the patients are healing twice as fast. Using two teaspoons three times daily in the nebulizer, full recovery is being reported in as little as three days.

# URINARY TRACT INFECTIONS

In three case studies, doctors treated three people with urinary tract infections (UTI's). They had the people drink two teaspoons, three times daily of the 10 ppm Nano silver liquid. They reported that the patients showed signs of recovery in a little over three days and were deemed as fully recovered in an average of just over five days. These numbers are very close to a number of other people that have reported similar findings in using the 10 ppm Nano silver. I had one military doctor call and say that she had a three star general's wife who had been in the hospital for three months with a UTI. She said that the infection was caused by a multi-drug resistant form of E. coli, and that she had been on a full regimen of antibiotics which had not worked. The doctor asked us to send her some product by overnight mail. We did so and she used the 10 ppm Nano silver in combination with the antibiotics. The doctor reported that the general's wife was able to fully recover from the infection within a week and she called us angels of mercy. I have found that with UTI's it may sometimes be necessary to take a larger dose of the liquid at one time to jumpstart the killing of the infecting bacteria. A number of doctors as well, have also reported faster results having their patients drink 4 ounces of the 10 ppm Nano silver twice daily for two days, and then cutting back to the two teaspoons three times daily until the infection is resolved.

# VAGINAL ODOR

The 10 ppm Nano silver liquid can be used as a douche to kill odor causing bacteria. The 24 ppm Nano silver gel can also be effectively used to kill odor causing bacteria. The gel can be applied with a vaginal applicator (5 ml.) or the gel can be inserted by being used as personal lubricant. Either way, bringing the gel in direct contact with the odor causing bacteria will have a very beneficial effect on the elimination of the odor and also the possible associated itch. The gel has also been safety tested and was found not to significantly disrupt the good or probiotic bacteria that helps protect the vaginal tract from pathogens.

## VAGINAL YEAST INFECTION

The 24 ppm Nano silver gel was reported to eliminate yeast infections in just 90 minutes of contact time by a major health magazine [13]. The woman's doctor and author, suggested that by putting a dime sized dob (3–5 ml) of the gel on a tampon and then inserting it into the vagina, the gel could eliminate the Candida infection within the 90 minutes. Doctors have also suggested that by using the gel as a personal lubricant, that the gel could help eliminate the yeast on both partners at the same time. It has also been reported that continued use of the 24 ppm Nano silver gel as a personal lubricant may help keep the woman from suffering yeast infections in the future. There is also mounting evidence that the gel can help kill or eliminate other vaginal pathogens and possibly STD's as well. Women have reported that the gel can also help eliminate both vaginal odor and itch. Vaginal probiotic studies showed that the 24 ppm Nano silver gel would do no significant damage to the good flora that lines and helps protect the vagina.

## WARTS

Warts are caused by virus and silver will many times have a very positive effect on them. The problem is getting the silver to the virus. Many warts have a hard skin coating on top which often times blocks the silvers ability to get to the actual virus. There are a number of ways to use silver to help get rid of the wart. One of the best is to use a product like Compound W etc., to strip the dead tissue off the top of the wart, then saturate a cotton ball with the 10 ppm Nano silver liquid and either hold it on the wart or tape the cotton ball in place for 10-30 minutes making sure it stays wet for the whole time. Repeat the process two to three times daily. Many people see positive results in just 3-7 days. In extreme cases I have heard of people injecting the liquid Nano silver directly into and around the wart with a small syringe, putting the silver in direct contact with the virus, but this should only be done under the direction of a doctor.

## WATER PURIFICATION

Two independent tests completed at a water purification laboratory, concluded that the 10 ppm Nano silver liquid would kill 100% of the natural and added bacteria in the raw river test water, in about 1.5 minutes of contact time, at a level of only 0.10 ppm (100 ppb's). That is a dilution of one to a hundred. One ounce of silver product put directly into 100 ounces of water etc. This means that one 8 ounce bottle of 10 ppm Nano-silver liquid would treat 6.25 gallons of water for bacteria or 0.78 gallons per ounce of the silver product. Water treatment works best with non-chlorinated water, and also water that has had the large organic material removed with a two micron backpacking or other similar filter. A good backpacking filter will filter out the large stuff (like giardia and crypto) but unfortunately will not remove bacteria from raw water. So by using both a backpacking filter and the 10 ppm Nano silver liquids, water treatment can be a reality almost anywhere a person goes. That also means that if you are traveling to another country and buy a 24 ounce bottled water, that you would need to add about two teaspoons of the silver product and wait about 1.5 minutes to drink the water, the silver should help kill any bacteria that may be in the bottled water.

# REFERENCES

1. David A. Revelli, June 18, 1999. Brigham Young University. Nano Silver vs. three commercial colloids.

2. Merck Manual, 18th Edition, pages 2021-2022, Toxic Nephoropathy or Heavy Metal Poisoning.

3. U. S. EPA Registration Eligibility Document for silver (RED Document), Page 2-3

4. Rustum Roy, M. Richard Hoover, A.S. Bhalla, Tania Slawecki, et al., Ultradilute Ag-Aquasols with extraordinary bactericidal properties: the role of the system Ag-0-H2O, Current Science Investigation 2007.

5. David A. Revelli, C. G. Lydiksen, J. D. Smith, R. W. Leavitt, A unique Silver Sol with braod antimicrobial properites, JSHO Vol 3 April 2011

6. A. De Souza, D. Mehta, R. W. Leavitt, Bactericidal activity of combinations of Silver-Water Dispersion with 19 antibiotics against seven microbial strains, Current Science. NO. &. October 2006

7. Holladay et al., United States Patent No.: 7,135,195 B2, Treatment Of Humans With Colloidal Silver Composition, November 14, 2006

8. G. Pedersen, B. M. Hedge, Silver Sol completely removes malaria parasites from the blood of human subjects infected with malaria in an average of five days, The Indian Practitioner, Vol. 63 September 2010

9. G. Pedersen, Effect of prophylactic treatment with ASAP-AGX-32 and ASAP Solutions on an avian influenza A (H5N1) virus infection in mice, JSHO August 17, 2008. Note-HIV data is the editor's note at the first of the article.

10. G. Pedersen, Keith Moeller, Silver Sol improves wound healing: Case studies in the use of silver sol in closing wounds (Including MRSA), preventing infection, inflammation and activating stem cells

11. Sheri C. Patel Research Centre, Oral Mouse Model Tests at 50, 500, 5000 mg/kg

12. Nichols, NAMSA ,Toxicity Tests, - 200 times normal adult dosage, July 7, 1999

13. Dr. Sherrill Sellman, A Silver Lining for Women's Health. Total Health Magazine. Volume 30,No. 5 Pg. 24-26.

14. J. R. Morones-Ramirez, J.A. Winkler, C.S. Spina, J.J. Collins. Silver Enhances Antibiotic Activity Against Gram Negative Bacteria. Sci. Transl. Med. 19 June 2013, Vol. 5, Issue 190.

15. The antibiotic crisis, News Nine, THE WEEK. November 22, 2013

16. U.S. CDC Website Http://www.cdc.gov/hai/organizms/cre. Info on Carbapenem-resistant Enterobactereriaceae or CRE.

17. William D. Moeller, U.S. Subcommittee on Africa Global Human Rights and International Operations. Committee on International Relations House of Representatives. April 26, 2005. Malaria and TB: Implementing Proven Treatment and Eradication Methods. Written testimony on Malaria

18. BYU, David A. Revelli, Silver in Glass vs. Plastic Containers. 2003.

19. Munger MA., Radwanski P., Hadlock GC., Stoddard G., Shaaban A., Falconer J.,Deering-Rice CE., Nanomedicine, June 28, 2013. In vivo human time-exposure study of orally dosed commercial silver Nano Particles

20. Smock Jk. Schmidt RL. Hadlock G. Stoddard G. Grainger DW. Munger MA. Assessment of orally dosed commercial silver Nanoparticles on human ex vivo platelet aggregation. May 2, 2013. University of Utah

21. R. Robinson, 2003. Bactericidal activity of ASAP Silver Solution on Yersinia Pestis, the etiological agent of plague. Department of Microbiology, Brigham Young University

22. A. Hafkine, 2003. ASAP antiviral activity in Hepatitis B; DNA Polymerase Inhibition, Reverse Transcriptase Inhibition. Hafkine Institute for Training, Research and Testing.

23. G. Pedersen, A fighting Chance. 2008. Pg. 57

24. Pedersen G. Silver Sol and the Successful Treatment of Hospital Acquired MRSA in Human Subjects with Ongoing Infection. Anti-Aging Therapeutics, Vol. 11, Chapter 35, pgs. 295-300.

25. C.G. Laboratories, April 8, 2010. Antimicrobial Time Kill Study Report. Eight pathogens including; Candida a., MRSA, VRE, etc. Challenge levels of 1-3 billion pathogens/ml. 90%+ kills at 5 min, at 10, 20, 30 ppm levels.

26. Nelson Labs - June 10, 2005. Antimicrobial testing – Hard surface. Kill times against Candida a., Trichophyten m., Aspergillus n., and Stachybotrys c., a type of black mold.

27. FDA ASAP Wound Dressing Gel- date cleared 04/02/09

28. Viridis BioPharma – March 2003- June 2003, Cytotoxicity of ASAP 10 and 22 ppm against both a Vero cell line and also a Hep2 cell line

29. Ron W. Leavitt Ph.D., February 18, 2009. SilverSol prevents Microorganisms from Becoming Resistant, a Discussion.